Finding Balance

Fitness and Training
for a Lifetime in Dance

Finding Balance

Fitness and Training
for a Lifetime in Dance

GIGI BERARDI

Dance Horizons/
Princeton Book Company, Publishers
Princeton, NJ

Directory of Selected Dance/Arts Medicine Clinics © 1990 by Jan Dunn.
Studio photograph of Risa Steinberg by David Fullard on cover. Courtesy of the
photographer.

A Dance Horizons Book
Princeton Book Company, Publishers
POB 57
Pennington, NJ 08534

Interior design by Anne O'Donnell
Cover design by Diana Coe

Library of Congress Cataloging-in-Publication Data

Berardi, Gigi M.
Finding balance : fitness and training for a lifetime in dance / Gigi Berardi.
    p.   cm.
"Dance horizons."
Includes bibliographical references (p.) and index.
ISBN 0-87127-160-5
1. Dancing.   2. Dancers.   3. Physical fitness.   4. Dancing—Accidents and
injuries—Prevention.   5. Health.   I. Title.
GV1595.B47   1991
792.8—dc20
                                                            90-52899

In loving memory

Jeff Duncan
(1930–1989)

Hank Gathers
(1967–1990)

Contents

List of Tables

List of Figures

Acknowledgments

I acknowledge the following individuals for their time, advice, and support in the initial phases of this project: Ruth Solomon, Richard Bachrach, Theresa Roberts, Robert Stephens, Suzanne Gordon, Mimi Moorehead, and Steven Scheck. For answering questions about specific material, I am grateful to Alex Dubé, Leonard Calabrese, Karen Clippinger-Robertson, Jay Cooper, John Garhammer, Leonard Leibowitz, Marika Molnar, Martha Myers, Jerome Schnitt, Diana Schnitt, Jay Seals, Carol Teitz, Ann McNeil, and Ellen Wallach.

I am grateful to the following for their careful and sensitive reading of numerous drafts of this manuscript and for their many helpful suggestions: Diana Cummins, Lovisa Josephson, Darrel Ramsey, Anandha Ray, Jan Dunn, Judy Gantz, Daniel Nagrin, Richard Braver, Arlene Levin, Robin Chmelar, and L.M. Vincent. Kenneth Laws and Zbigniew Przasnyski deserve special mention for their critical review and editing of the manuscript. Thanks also to Richard Carlin for encouragement and support in this project, and for his editorial work. And at Princeton Book Company, I thank Charles Woodford, publisher, and Debi Elfenbein, editor. I also thank Lovisa Josephson for writing the detailed medical and dance glossaries, and Auralie Logan for her skillful indexing. Numerous hours of work were required to produce the glossaries and index; for their time and expertise I am grateful. I am especially thankful to Barbara Palfy for copyediting the manuscript. For her masterful editing and patience, I am especially grateful.

Others who have helped me in various ways and who I should like to thank are Judith Carney, Nancy Lee, Lei Li, Judy Roberts, Judy Scalin, Kathleen Schiller, Allan Ryan, Selma Jeanne Cohen, Erianne Aichner, Elaine Dalrymple, Cindy DiBenedetti, Liisa Gardner, Leslie Getz, Michael Heiman, Paula Bourla, Janice Gudde Plastino, Linda Kelly, Rachelle Katz, Dora Sowden, Arline Miller, Don Bradburn, Arne Youngerman, Jan Gal, Lisa Fusillo, Antoinette Marich, Michael Schreiber, and Bert Mandelbaum; and at UCLA: Judith Alter, Angelia Leung, Carol Scothorn, Allegra Fuller Snyder, Elsie Dunin, Emma Lewis Thomas, Judith Mitoma, Doris Siegel, Ellen Sinatra, Stephanie Schoelzel, Silvily Kessler-Thomas, Alma Hawkins, Roslyn Moore, Wendy Temple, James Allaway, and Sam Jones.

Special thanks is given to all the movement teachers who inspired this work, knowingly or unknowingly: Jan Hyatt, Margaret Hills, Alix Keast, Karen Bell, Janice Kovar, Saga Ambegaokar, Bill Evans, Elizabeth Walton, Susan Matheke, Anna de Boisson, Joyce Morgenroth, and especially Jeff Duncan, to whom this book is dedicated. Jeff was a teacher, mentor, and colleague who refused to compromise his integrity or his craft—whether for a university position, for commercial success, or for anyone's approval.

Thanks to the photographers whose work is used in this book, from whom every effort has been made to obtain permission:

Peter Affeld
Jay Anderson
A. Pierce Bounds
Richard T. Braver, D.P.M.
Tom Brazil
Steven Caras
Tom Caravaglia
Robin Chmelar
Dennis Deloria
Jed Downhill
Kenn Duncan
Johan Elbers
James Fry
David Fullard
Anthony Hall
Martha Kalman

Daniel Kramer
Gilles Larrain
Megan Lawrence
John Lindquist
Herbert Migdoll
Marika Molnar, P.T.
Julyen Norman
Bill Owen
Wm. J. Reilly
Mike Sands
Phyllis Steele
Leslie Sternlieb
Carol C. Teitz, M.D.
Cylla von Tiedemann
Weiferd Watts
Tom Wilson

In addition, the following companies/institutions generously provided photographs: Merce Cunningham Dance Company, Dance Exchange, Dance Theatre Workshop, *The Dickinsonian,* Danny Grossman Dance Company, Erick Hawkins Dance Company, Joffrey Ballet, Margalit Marshall Dance, Mark Morris Dance, and Robbins Inc.

Thanks also to the following dancers and health professionals who posed for the photographs: Karah Abiog, Victor Barbee, Cathleen Fischbach, Barbara Gagas, Judy Gantz, Jerel Hilding, Kathryn Karipides, Louis Kavouras, Kenneth Laws, Valerie Madonia, Peter Marshall, Cathy Paine, and Angela Patrinos.

Sincere thanks is extended to the many dancers interviewed over the past three years; it is their comments that provided the basis for related articles and for this narrative. Their cooperation is greatly appreciated. The following is only a partial list:

Merrill Ashley	Murray Louis
Karen Bell	Adam Luders
Oleg Briansky	Margalit Marshall
Trisha Brown	Bruce Marks
Richard Colton	Patricia McBride
Carmen de Lavallade	Kevin McKenzie
Daniel Duell	John Meehan
June Finch	Phoebe Neville
Judith Fugate	Fayard Nicholas
Claudia Gitelman	Cathy Paine
Danny Grossman	Wendy Perron
Erick Hawkins	Tom Rawe
Jerel Hilding	Don Redlich
Kelly Holt	Keith Sabado
David Howard	Danny Shapiro
Jan Hyatt	Joanie Smith
Judith Jamison	Christine Spizzo
Kathryn Karipides	Risa Steinberg
Allegra Kent	Jennifer Way
David Landis	Patricia Wilde
Peggy Lawler	Lonna Wilkinson
Bella Lewitzky	Nina Weiner

My most sincere gratitude is extended to the many students I have taught, for their insights and optimism. And to one very special student, for his determination and conviction, and to whom also I dedicate this book—Hank Gathers. For having known this elite athlete, while I taught at Loyola Marymount University, and living his dream with him for just a little while, I am most grateful.

Gigi Berardi
Los Angeles, California

Preface:
Warm-up

"To retire to what? What do you do? Vegetate or reminisce or something? No—I want to exist now—in the moment."
                                   —Martha Graham, age 96[1]

Exist now—in the moment. For many in professional dance, it is hard to do just that. In 1983, McGraw-Hill published Suzanne Gordon's *Off Balance: The Real World of Ballet.* It is a penetrating study, the result of interviews with dancers in the companies of American Ballet Theatre, New York City Ballet, Pennsylvania Ballet, and others. What Suzanne Gordon found was a world of artists and would-be artists struggling for control over their bodies and their lives. For many, it was a losing battle.

Suzanne Gordon's book was a disturbing eye-opener for me. I had always been surrounded by teachers, many of whom were in their 40s and 50s, teaching modern and ballet technique classes, who continued to perform. I of course knew that many professionals stopped dancing in their 20s and 30s. What I couldn't understand was that this early "retirement age" was accepted as inevitable since there *are* dancers who are making a *career* out of dance, and they continue to perform. Their stories must be told, containing a message for young and old dancers alike: you don't have to be a 17-year-old anorexic in a professional school to be a dancer.

Much of my book is a reaction to the research and negative narrative that is published about dance—mostly classical ballet—in the United States. Thus, some of my discussion is directed specifically to classically trained dancers even though my critical writing and training affinities lie with both classical and modern dance forms.

Fortunately, modern dancers are being studied more. Martha Myers, Ruth Solomon, and others are pioneers of such research. In the second issue of the 1989–1990 volume of *Kinesiology and Medicine for Dance*, one of three articles on diet, nutrition, and weight management in dance dealt specifically with non-classically trained dance populations. Research agendas are changing—at least in terms of subjects with training other than in classical ballet. It's still the youthful dancers, however, who tend to be studied. They're the ones most visible at universities and in big-city professional dance companies. The dancers I interviewed for this book—in modern, ballet, and ethnic dance—were more than thirty years of age.

Although hundreds of dancers could have been interviewed, I focused on those who were more well known. It is true that most of the dancers I interviewed who were in their 40s and older tended to be modern dancers. It is also true that they don't represent everybody in dance. Not everyone is a Murray Louis or a Carmen de Lavallade. Nevertheless, there are people in their 40s still dancing in ballet companies, and similarly, in ethnic dance and show dance. These latter two areas of professional dance, however, I did not emphasize due to time and space constraints rather than inherent worthiness.

The dancers were forthcoming in their interviews, which I conducted formally and informally over the past three years. I realized that those dancers with no formal training in kinesiology— Jeff Duncan, Patricia McBride, Daniel Nagrin, and many others— were speaking from experience on what scientists and academicians deduced from systematic investigation. The dancers interviewed are *practicing* kinesiologists, and their stories and advice often—although not always—have a firm footing in dance science. What is clear is that this anecdotal information is usually every bit as sound as the "good science" appearing in refereed literature.

From these narratives, I have written the "Dancer Profiles." The reflections and comments in the profiles are related directly to the issues of performance, training, and technique discussed in the chapters. Inspired by their comments, I wrote text on the training, diet, and fitness issues that might confront a dancer in her or his training from age 17 to 77 and beyond.

This book contains an *overview* of pertinent training and fitness issues and findings that should be of interest to dancers and dance educators of all ages. It is not rife with blanket recommendations or recipes. The published literature provides no foundation for this when the research findings are so gray, i.e., being so highly qualified with caveats and disclaimers. How can one advocate one warm-up over another, one method of stretching, when the research findings (and questions asked) change so dramatically over time as new research and/or experience comes to light? Thus, I have provided a critical survey of the main issues and interpretations of research that make sense for dancers of the 1990s.

The target audience for this book is *not* the community of dance medicine and science scholars for which there are numerous journals and publications to challenge their ideas and stimulate their research programs. It is *not* academicians who teach courses on theory and write great books and serve on important committees. There are numerous scholarly books available for them. It is *not* editors of dance-related journals who are more interested in marking territory than writing on substantive issues.

The target audience for this book *is* professional dancers and students, as well as teachers, critics, historians, and audiences of professional dance. What I mean by "professional" dance is discussed at some length in Chapter 1.

The book has been organized into six chapters. There are dance and medical/technical glossaries for reference at the back of the book. Those readers with limited time or specific interests/backgrounds may want to read certain chapters.

Chapter 1 introduces the reader to the realities of professional dance. Chapter 2 presents an overview of injuries in dance, and lists conventional and alternative treatments. Chapter 3 emphasizes the physical analysis of dance technique, with the goal being avoidance of debilitating injury and prolonging professional careers.

Chapter 4 contains guidelines for fitness regimens. They have worked for people whom I respect, people who have been dancing for over 30 years. They may not work for everybody. Dance training and conditioning—and diet, discussed in Chapter 5—are ultimately very personal. However, dancers' taking control of their bodies and their lives must also be a very public act. Dancers must work together to challenge intolerable working conditions and constraining aesthetic norms as discussed in Chapter 6. Others have gone before us who have pioneered these changes. It is up to us to advance them.

— *One* —

Dance: A Demanding Profession

The image and presence of youth and thinness dominate much of the dance world. In classical ballets, dancers portray willowy princes and fair maidens, the young just barely coming of age, the newly wed and the newly dead. In abstract works, youthful dancers' shiny Lycra unitards emphasize protruding pelvic bones and ribs (Fig. 1); bodies are streamlined rather than robust. This look is changing—slowly.[1]

Some dancers virtually risk their lives for their art. They push themselves too much, they work too hard—sacrificing friends, family, food, sleep, not to mention reasonable income. Not only is professional dance emotionally and physically demanding, but also employment is short-lived. Realistically, dancers often consider it an occupation rather than a career, since the opportunities for advancement or promotion are so limited. In ballet, if dancers haven't made it to soloist or principal status by the time they've reached age twenty-five or thirty, it's unlikely they ever will.

But trend is not destiny. Despite public expectations and physical constraints, dancers are dancing into their thirties, and forties, and far beyond. In order to do this, they must make decisions on how they train and how they can care for injuries, which are often emphasized in "how-to" books, and will be considered at length in Chapters 2 through 5. Even more important determinants of career longevity are what and where dancers are willing to dance. These, discussed in Chapter 6, must

1

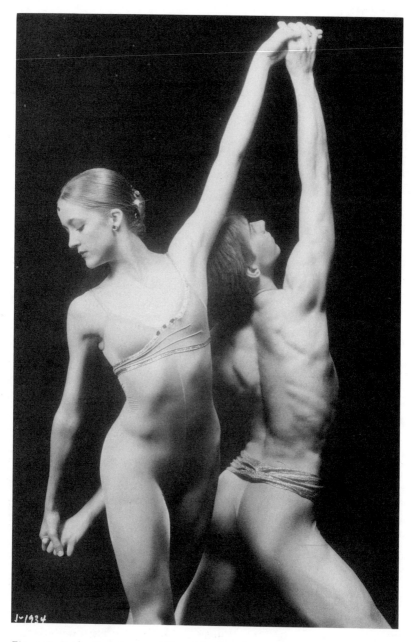

Figure 1. Leslie Carothers and Tom Mossbrucker. Carothers epitomizes the sylphlike classical ballerina. *(Photo by Herbert Migdoll. Courtesy of The Joffrey Ballet.)*

be addressed aggressively by dance students, teachers, choreographers, artistic directors, scholars, and critics.

What follows is a survey for *all* dancers of injury prevention and effective treatment, of diet and conditioning, of training with good teachers. Ultimately, dancers must find a balance between training and performance, body image and nutritional imperatives, injury treatment and performance schedules, dance aesthetics and dance kinesiology—what is considered aesthetically pleasing and what is structurally/functionally possible—as well as personal needs and professional goals. Only then will dancers be empowered to take control of their lives and make professional dance a career.

The experiences of the dancers who have found such a balance in their professional lives are presented in profiles at the end of each chapter. Reading them, dancers everywhere and of all ages may be encouraged to acknowledge some of the harsh realities of the profession—intense physical demands, relentless work schedules, obsession with youth and thinness—not so much to deny as to refuse to be limited by them.

The Show Must Go On

Few professional sports can compare with dance in terms of the relentless demands placed on the mind and body. Although cyclists race at close to maximum capacity and baseball pitchers put stress on the highly mobile shoulder joint to the physical limit, causing injuries, soreness, fatigue, and inflammation, "dancers, ranked with elite athletes in terms of their need to compete and perform regardless of injury and pain, are never supposed to show that pain."[2]

Dance is not seasonal and dancers do not stop dancing with most injuries—they can't. One of the dancer's biggest fears is of being "sidelined" and replaced. They simply can't afford to miss an opportunity to perform, especially in a featured role. Their career is at stake. Even their companies may be at stake because many modern dance and small ballet companies have no understudies. The dancers know that the company depends on them; they don't want to have a reputation of unreliability, of "always being injured." So, they perform. Friends are telling them they can do it and medical professionals are helping them to do it.[3] Perhaps this is how one explains the classic example of young Robert Weiss of New York City Ballet (NYCB) who snapped his Achilles tendon during a performance, yet continued to dance. Eventually, the pain became intolerable.

Most of the time, the audience is oblivious to the pain and injuries that dancers suffer, and the show must and often does go on. The soloist landing from a grand allegro jump may actually be suffering from ankle tendinitis or debilitating arthritis in the knees. A premier danseur may perform with multiple stress fractures in his lower leg. Mikhail Baryshnikov's inflamed foot is hardly noticeable in *Coppélia*.[4] Rudolf Nureyev dances strapped in tape up to the middle of his thigh. Danny Grossman, who describes himself as "in trouble from the waist down," danced for Paul Taylor for ten years without missing one performance.

One dancer I interviewed had fractured her heel bone during a performance, splintering the bone into chips. She should have rested, stopped dancing. But telling dancers to stop dancing means that the person giving the advice knows nothing about professional dance.

Only one week may be all that is necessary to recover from an ankle sprain, shinsplints, or a mild muscle bruise, but one week to a dancer may seem like forever. Even worse, sometimes complete bed rest is indicated. How is complete bed rest possible? The rent must be paid, classes must be taught, someone has to buy and prepare food. The dancer just makes do, maybe with a little ice, certainly with a lot of antiswelling/pain medication.[5]

The good news is that with the advent of specialists in dance medicine, many dancers do not have to stop dancing when injured. Instead, they can *selectively* rest body parts—especially when the upper body is the affected area—and limit certain movements. This is only justified after examination of the injured body part and factors causing the injury. The specialist may recommend use of a soft cast, modifications in technique, or flexibility/strengthening exercises, all of which enable the dancer to continue activity during recovery of certain injuries (see Chapter 2 for further discussion).

Performance Schedules

What I've described above is the private drama dancers live as they try to meet demanding performance schedules in spite of injury and pain. Just how much dancing do typical performance schedules require? When is the work too much? Artistic director Oleg Briansky warns, "Dancers work too much—eight performances in a week. You don't allow horses to run eight times in one week."[6]

Former American Ballet Theatre (ABT) principal John Meehan performed in 260 performances of the musical *Song and Dance* in one year. In a personal interview, NYCB principal Merrill Ashley noted that at one time she was dancing "nightly performances of sometimes two and even three ballets."[7] She admitted that "there were probably lots of little things that flared up." Later, when she danced only four to five times each week there were fewer injuries. Other principal dancers—especially NYCB's seasoned males—are not in such a comfortable position that they can determine their own work schedules. For dancers in the corps, there is simply no choice—they dance every night.

Obviously, there are huge differences in the performance schedules within and among dance companies. For example, in seven performances of the Joffrey Ballet (during one week of a four-week season in May 1989 at the Los Angeles Music Center), the dancers were scheduled to perform in the following number of ballets out of a possible twenty-four:

Mary Barton	11	Meg Gurin	8
Cameron Basden	10	Julie Janus	11
Linda Bechtold	7	Tina LeBlanc	8
Leslie Carothers	7	Valerie Madonia	8
Jill Davidson	11	Elizabeth Parkinson	11
Deborah Dawn	8	Victoria Pasquale	11
Jodie Gates	7	Beatriz Rodriguez	9
Charlene Gehm	7	Kim Sagami	15
Cynthia Giannini	11	Lissette Salgado	4
Kathryn Ginden	9	Johanna Snyder	5
	Carole Vallesky	8	

Patrick Corbin	11	Peter Narbutas	16
Carl Corry	10	Brent Phillips	7
Glenn Edgerton	11	Roger Plaut	12
Glen Harris	5	Joseph Schnell	6
Jerel Hilding	9	Adam Sklute	6
Douglas Martin	14	Edward Stierle	9
Edward Morgan	6	Tyler Walters	14
Tom Mossbrucker	10	Ashley Wheater	7
	Mark Wuest	9	

It is difficult to compare the rigor of performance schedules of individual dancers. Using the example above, some of the dancers were featured in the ballets (Leslie Carothers, Tina LeBlanc, Beatriz Rodriguez, Carole Vallesky, Glenn Edgerton, Ashley Wheater), whereas others danced primarily supporting roles.[8] Leslie Carothers and Linda Bechtold each danced in seven ballets, yet Carothers had mostly principal roles.

The length and choreography of ballets are also factors in the demands placed on dancers. Frederick Ashton's *Monotones II* requires extreme flexibility of its ballerina (Elizabeth Parkinson in the first week of the 1989 season at the Music Center); Gerald Arpino's *Valentine* requires greater dramatic flair and intensity (danced by Beatriz Rodriguez and Glenn Edgerton in the Los Angeles performances). Balanchine's reconstructed *Cotillon* is an ensemble piece that asks for camaraderie more than batterie—it is engaging for its choreography, rather than for virtuosity. Nevertheless, the more one dances as part of an ensemble or corps, the more likely the chance of injury. Landing more solo roles might be the best way to prolong a career, but there are no guarantees.

Another way to prolong a career is to avoid heavy touring schedules. This is unrealistic, of course, for many dance companies; touring is often mandated by financial exigencies and obligations. Company directors know that heavy touring schedules are a risk, as much for the dancer's health as the company's solvency.[9] Nevertheless, the risk is usually taken. The travels of two modern dance companies are not untypical: in one year, Twyla Tharp's and Erick Hawkins's companies each visited and performed in twenty-six cities in the United States and abroad. Touring and all that it involves—constant travel, fatigue, new and sometimes inadequate accommodations, unresilient stage floors, no time to rehearse, virtually no time to eat, little to eat except fast foods, adjusting to different drinking water,[10] being away from family and friends—are a reality of life for most dancers in professional companies. It is not uncommon to hear dancers talk of quitting just to get off the touring circuit.

It is important for younger dancers to see just how demanding the rehearsal and performance regimens are in major professional companies. They have to be aware that there are other employment opportunities in dance—for example, in academic and community institutions—in which performance is not the sole source of income and, typically, performance schedules are not so rigorous. A case in point is a small Ohio dance company that performed approximately 100 times over ten years within the state.

To be a performer does not necessarily involve performing every night, especially if one is interested in longevity. There are many dancers who consider themselves performers, even though they're not on the road three months of each year. They dance at a college or high school, a church or barn, a community theatre or open park three or four or six times each year.[11] For them, performing with a company of national repute is not all-important. They, too, are performers, although not professional dancers in my use of the word.[12]

Overuse: Practice Does Not Make Perfect

Dancers try to achieve the near impossible. They work on the bigger, higher, and faster jump, 180-degree hip rotation for classical ballet turnout, the perfect landing from a double tour en l'air, clear execution of a double cabriole, and dazzling turns. The problem is that they often work on these steps too much—day in and day out.

If dancers could achieve perfection through repetition, critics would have nothing to write about. Dancers are champions at repeating movements; they get plenty of opportunity in daily class and rehearsals (see profile of Daniel Nagrin on page 29).

In order to improve, the dancer needs new information and insights into *how* the movement is performed. This must come from a teacher or from source material that the dancer respects. Some dancers are auditory learners, some are visual; some are kinesthetic and need to move to incorporate the correct placement for a given movement into their neuromuscular patterning. Some dancers are highly analytical and want to understand the mechanics of the movements they perform. Dancers have to be aggressive in seeking out the *how* in ways of learning with which they are comfortable: how to find balance when turning? how to create the illusion of floating in the air? how to increase the height of leg extension?

Repetition is not enough. Of course it's important to practice movement, but not if dancers have structural anomalies that prevent its correct execution. Not if they are making harmful compensations for limited muscle flexibility. Not if they are clueless about what muscles need to be strengthened before a movement can be sustained. According to Erick Hawkins, "You don't practice, practice; you practice *theory*, based on principles of kinesiology." This assumes a working and practical knowledge of some form of movement principles (see Chapter 3 for a full discussion).

Injuries are caused by dancers' repeated attempts to force their bodies beyond anatomical limitations. For example, a movement

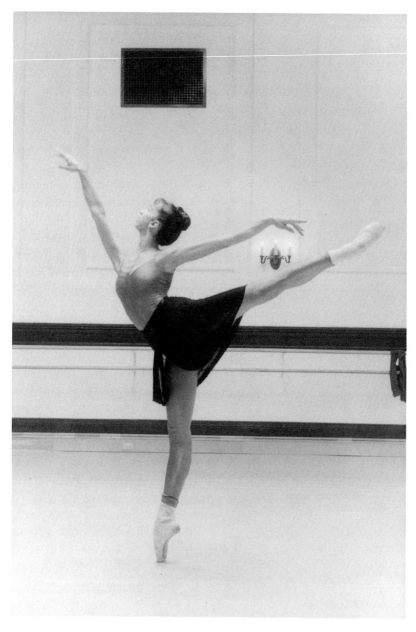

Figure 2. A long lower extremity can act as a powerful lever on the lower back, where the force may not be dissipated widely owing to the short torso (see Allan J. Ryan and Robert E. Stephens, *Dance Medicine*, p. 22). Here, Valerie Madonia of The Joffrey Ballet poses in an arabesque. *(Photo by Weiferd Watts)*

such as extending the thigh at the hip in an arabesque exacerbates the forces on the lower spine, especially when the torso is short (Fig. 2). Eventually, the chronic stress on the body results in premature deterioration of connective tissue in the pelvic and lower spine areas.

Examples of Overuse Injuries

Repeated jumps and leaps on unresilient dance surfaces eventually take their toll on the dancer's body. This would not be so much a problem if protective footwear was worn (which it is not) and proper alignment of the lower body when landing was used.

Table 1 gives examples of common overuse injuries in dance. What is responsible for the injuries? The factors—all of which will be discussed in later chapters—are usually the same: repeated dancing on unresilient dance surfaces; poor technique; pathogenic choreography; anatomical limitations; muscle imbalance; and returning to dance before adequate recovery of an injury.

Table 1. Examples of Different Types of Overuse Injuries and Some of Their Causes*

Type of Injury

   Stress fractures of the metatarsal bones of the foot
   Plantar fasciitis and strain of the plantar fascia
   Achilles tendinitis
   Shinsplints

Possible Causes

   Repeated jumps and leaps, unresilient dance surfaces
   Excessive pronation (feet rolling in)
   Excessive eversion (feet rolling out, sickling)
   Forcing turnout
   Choreography (e.g., ball-to-heel "stage running," allowing minimal
       contact with the floor when landing)
   Structural (e.g., tight, narrow tendons)
   Improper technique (resulting, e.g., in a weakened quadriceps muscle)
   Inadequate warm-up (this is a contributing factor to most injuries)

*The information in this table, discussed at greater length in Chapter 2, is from Stuart Wright, *Dancer's Guide to Injuries of the Lower Extremity: Diagnosis, Treatment, and Care* (New York: Cornwall Books, 1985). Wright's book is highly recommended to dancers interested in making their own diagnoses of dance injuries and developing appropriate treatment plans.

For example, to protect against stress fractures of the metatarsals, proper technique is essential. Dancers who land from jumps with their big toes lifted (this is done to avoid rolling-in of the foot) are prone to stress fractures, commonly of the second metatarsal.

Painful inflammation of the plantar fascia of the foot, Achilles tendinitis, and shinsplints can also be attributed to poor technique or inherited structural malalignment. Dancers who land with their "heel up" (i.e., with the heel of the foot failing to make contact with the floor) suffer chronic injury. Unfortunately, this describes many dancers. Dancers with shallow plié, weak quadriceps, or weak feet are going to have problems rolling through the entire foot when landing in fast-tempo ballets.[13] If the floor is not allowed to absorb the shock from landing—which can be easily triple or quadruple the forces that pass through the foot and ankle—something must, and usually it is the soft tissues of the body, with shock finally transmitted to the bone.

In sum, repeated landings from aerial work can result in microtears to tendons and in chronic inflammation. The name of the game is shock absorption and dancers don't know how to begin to play it. What is a dancer to do?

Shock Absorption

DANCE FOOTWEAR

A contributing factor to overuse injury is the lack of protective footwear. Other athletes use some kind of protective footwear, but dance, which is much more athletic now than in the days of Isadora Duncan, still uses shoes that are not.

Figures 3 and 4 show the footwear worn in ballet. Ballet slippers are soft, flexible, and are usually made of canvas or leather. Pointe shoes are more rigid, the toe being "blocked" (i.e., stiffened with glue).[14] Neither shoe offers shock absorption from aerial work.

Aesthetically, the effect of the pointe shoe is stunning. It helps to extend the long line of the body when the foot is raised from the floor and it facilitates the execution of multiple pirouettes.[15] But for aerial work it is a liability, providing little shock absorption. In a recent interview, Merrill Ashley is quoted to complain about the hopping on pointe required by the Petipa choreography in *Sleeping Beauty*, which she performs.[16] Depending on the shock absorption properties of the flooring that night, most of the impact is being absorbed by her knees, hips, and spine. This is true in general when any aerial work is performed in the pointe shoe.

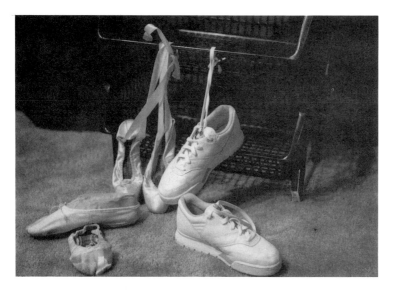

Figure 3. Both the soft ballet slippers (*left foreground*) and the rigid pointe shoes (*left background*) have no shock absorption properties. The shock-absorbing qualities of the "athletic" shoe (*right*) are given mostly by the innersole, midsole, and outsole of the shoe. The midsole and outsole materials must not be so thick as to prevent full range of motion of the metatarsals. *(Photo by Richard Braver, D.P.M.)*

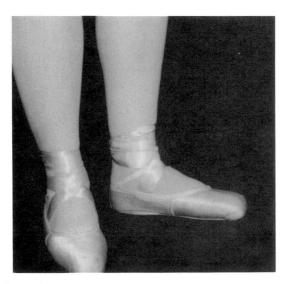

Figure 4. Pointe shoes with blocked toe. *(Photo by Carol Teitz, M.D.)*

Things may be bad in ballet, but they're even worse in modern dance, for which usually no shoes are worn. This is in keeping with the original ideology of modern dance: freedom in movement and expressiveness, unrestricted by clothing. Unfortunately, the biomechanics of movement at work in contemporary choreography does not reflect this ideology. For today's modern dancers, it's much safer to wear athletic shoes, as in Danny Grossman's work (see profile, page 27). This makes sense for *some* dancers, for *some* choreography. It works for his choreographic aesthetics (Fig. 5). In addition to providing shock absorption, the athletic shoe also provides lateral and hindfoot stability. Turns, however, must be carefully negotiated—or avoided—to prevent abrupt, twisting movements that might damage the cartilage in the knee.

Dance Flooring

Hard, unresilient floors can easily ruin a dancer's career. According to Jay Seals, an expert on flooring surfaces for dance, "Dance professionals . . . regard the dance floor [for resiliency and shock absorption] as one of the most important variables (second to physical conditioning) affecting performance."[17] Studies are needed, however, on the actual external and internal forces acting on the dancer's body upon impact with the floor.

Many injuries of the lower leg, such as shinsplints, inflammation of the tendons of the ankle, and stress fractures of the foot and leg, may be directly attributed to dancing on a too hard surface. Likewise, surfaces too soft can lead to increased fatigue and chronic injury: a soft dance surface requires the dancer to push off harder for jumps because it has too much "give" and too little resiliency. In addition, if the dancer has structural imbalances, such as a rolled-in arch, landing from a jump on a soft surface will exaggerate the potentially harmful movements resulting from the imbalance. This is because the ground reactive forces are decreased and the flooring is not acting quickly to stop the excessive motions.

It is almost impossible to control the dance environment, especially when a company is touring (unless specified previously in a contract). When ABT tours, they carry their own portable floor—a suspended dance-floor system, consisting of synthetic material and void-free plywood. It can be laid over any floor that is structurally sound, including a concrete slab. It is generally agreed that there is a lower incidence of impact injuries when suspended dance-floor systems are used.

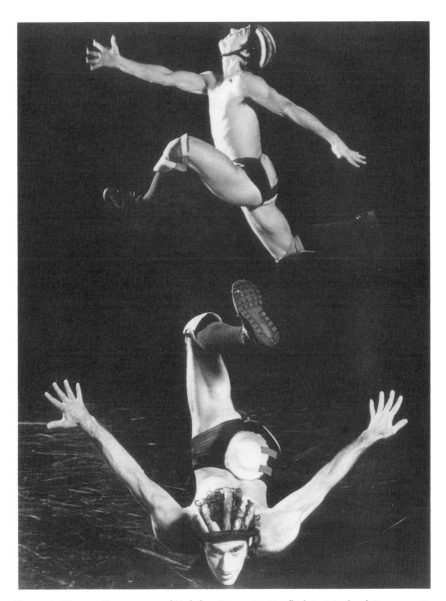

Figure 5. Danny Grossman and Bohdan Romaniw (in flight). Much of Grossman's choreography allows the dancers to wear athletic shoes. *(Photo by Cylla von Tiedemann. Courtesy of the Danny Grossman Dance Company.)*

Dancers and artistic directors alike must be educated on what is acceptable construction for dance floors and then make decisions as to whether or not, and how, they will perform. Dancers must take the responsibility of evaluating the performance environment, although how that can be done without expensive measuring instruments remains a problem. Friction can be determined by dancing on the floor; "give" is more difficult. Kenneth Laws (see profile, page 95) suggests that "what is needed is something like a standard steel ball, to be dropped from a height of four feet. The height of the bounce can then be measured."[18] This at least mimics the relative "give" of a dance floor.

Studies have been conducted and standard test methods determined for characterizing flooring designs (Fig. 6a). The test methods include ASTM 355-78 Dynamic Shock Test, the Japanese International Standard, and the DIN Standard. For example, the principal DIN standard criteria that combine to form a dance floor's overall comfort, safety, and performance include shock absorption (the floor's ability to reduce the impact force of the dancer), standard vertical deformation (deflection of the floor along the vertical axis upon impact), and sliding characteristics (measurement of the surface friction of the finished floor surface; this test simulates a dancer's sliding and rotational movements).

Ideally, a floor should have some "give," but should neither deform permanently under pressure, be excessively springy, nor be rigid. The Permacushion® Sleeper System manufactured by Robbins uses ⅝-inch rubber pads placed underneath the wooden boards (sleepers) to provide varying degrees of shock absorption and resiliency (Figs. 6b–c). The SpringAire® ballet floor system features leveling blocks—special spring coils attached to 2 × 4-inch sleepers approximately every ten inches along the sleeper (Fig. 6d).

Pushing the Body Image

Audiences want their dancers slender and svelte. Critics bristle at the sight of a male dancer's exposed midriff slightly extending over his dance belt. Many artistic directors are manic about their dancers' weight and shape. The worst critic of all—the mirror—invites an obsession with body image that would put top-dollar fashion models to shame. What does all this add up to? An obsession with thinness of Herculean proportion.

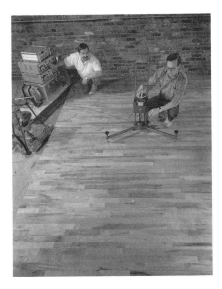

Figure 6a. Permacushion® Sleeper System: Testing for standard vertical deformation and deflective indentation. *(Photo courtesy of the Robbins Company.)*

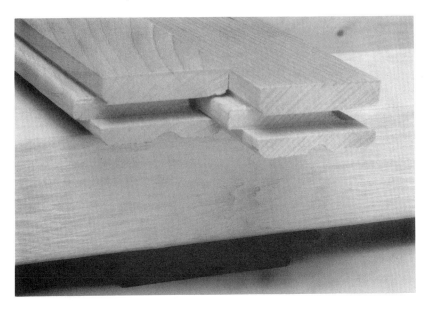

Figure 6b. Permacushion® Sleeper System: ⅝-inch pads. *(Photo courtesy of the Robbins Company.)*

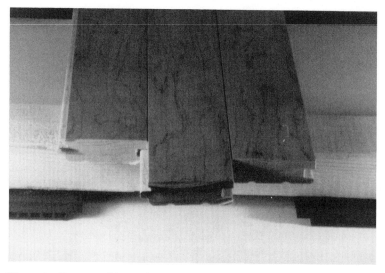

Figure 6c. Permacushion® Sleeper System: ⅝-inch pads. *(Photo courtesy of the Robbins Company.)*

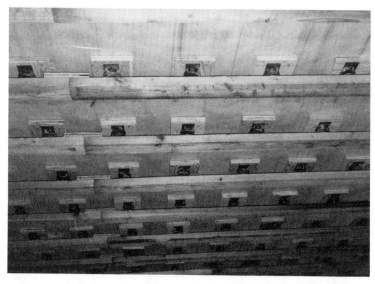

Figure 6d. SpringAire® Underlayment System. *(Photo courtesy of the Robbins Company.)*

Dancers graciously indulge in the obsession. And thus the dance world is populated with the thin, trim, and lean. But "thin" is relative; dancers are fixated on being very thin. In the battle for critics' superlatives, they have a fighting chance to win this one at least.

But there comes a point when dancers must stop pushing the image to its limits and listen to their body.[19] Often, it is older or more mature dancers who feel that they can afford to do this. Not to ease off, though, results in chronic injury—and perhaps permanent disability. A case in point is Michelle Benash (formerly of ABT) who is virtually crippled from her early days of dancing. This she attributes partially to excessive dieting when she was young. Poor eating habits in general—dieting, low carbohydrate intake—lead to fatigue and possible injury. This is probably what Benash is referring to when she mentions her knee problems:

> When I was young I ruined my body. . . . It wasn't just the dancing that did it; it was the dieting. You were supposed to be thin, super thin, so I starved myself. I lived on 300 calories a day. . . . I know my knee problem is related to all that.[20]

What Benash describes is self-induced starvation, resembling the symptoms of anorexia nervosa, "ballet's dirty little secret." It is not just ballet's secret. Although in general modern dancers don't aspire to the skeletal look rife in ballet, the desire to be thin—the job requirement to be thin—and the eating disorders that make it possible are there. This is also true for Broadway, show, jazz, and tap dancers.

Anorexia nervosa (severe emaciation resulting from self-imposed weight loss), bulimia (compulsive eating, usually followed by self-induced vomiting), abusive use of cathartics (medicines that increase the rate of bowel evacuation), diuretics (agents that promote urination), and emetics (agents that promote vomiting) are well deserving of any and all attention they can receive in the scientific and popular literature. To this end, physician-author L. M. Vincent has written a particularly concise, thorough, and well-informed discussion of body image and eating disorders of dancers in *Competing with the Sylph*. Vincent discusses the enormous pressures on the dancer to conform to ideal weight, form, and age:

> There are plenty of reasons why dancers have to be thin, should one bother to ask. But there are many reasons why the aesthetic considerations of dance should not be given carte blanche. . . . Not that . . . there will be much of a market in the foreseeable future for obese ballet dancers; still, let us cast aside our biases

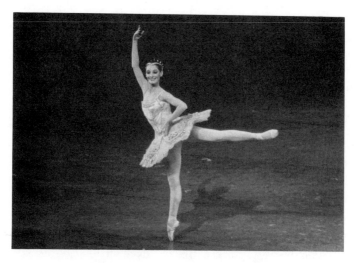

Figure 7a. Cynthia Gregory performing at the ABT gala in New York City in 1985. *(Photo by William J. Reilly)*

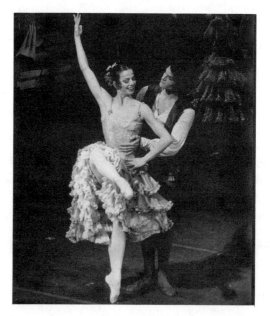

Figure 7b. ABT's Martine van Hamel with the late Patrick Bissell. *(Photo by William J. Reilly)*

(as well as our knowledge of the exigencies of the dance world today) and assume a broader perspective.[21]

The point is that the dance world, at least in some circles, is big enough to accommodate many body types. This is not to say that the specter of the "Balanchine" look—an "anorexic Peter Pan on *pointe*"[22]—no longer permeates the dance world, but there are alternative body types, notably among modern dancers and older ballet dancers (Fig. 7a–b).

Vincent continues:

> If you're intent upon performing (regardless of level), recognize and accept your physicality, and work within your abilities. Find a type of dance or company that your body is best suited for rather than attempting to overhaul your body.

Vincent is optimistic: competitive ballet schools are becoming a bit more lenient about weight in preprofessional levels; the health problems (gynecological and otherwise) associated with excessive thinness are receiving more attention in the literature.

Nevertheless, American ballet dancers are up against some apparent absolutes in the aesthetic of the slender body. One might even be able to quantify certain aspects of "smoothness of line" that involve length/width ratio of the body. There is no doubt that the aesthetics of dance (see Chapter 6) and the aesthetics of the dancer's size and shape must be reevaluated.

Perhaps we are going through an aesthetic "swing," a return to seeing and *appreciating* older and more full-bodied dancers on the stage. As Vincent observes:

> We are becoming older as a population, and the obsessive identification with youth may be waning. Feminist ideals have undoubtedly had a positive effect, not to mention the growing involvement of women in choreography. Role models are changing as well. . . . We recognize that adolescent gymnasts, despite their technical virtuosity, are not always able to pull off the artistic aspects of a program that require a greater element of maturity.

It is not just the ballet dancers who need to pull back, to ease off, from obsessive body image and/or work schedule. If the desire to dance is there and dancers truly want to continue to work, then men and women of all forms of dance must forge their own aesthetics, with confidence and perseverance. This won't come easily.

Older Dancers: So What About Retirement?

To the nondance population, "getting old" doesn't mean much in these days of vibrant middle-aged baby boomers and semiretired septuagenarians. Age, like thinness, is relative. People don't get old, they get older. What is clear is that the changes associated with aging (e.g., loss of strength, endurance, flexibility, and muscle mass) *accompany* aging rather than being *caused* by it—even in dance.

If only someone would tell this to dancers and their company managers, artistic directors, mentors, coaches, audiences, and so on. Many athletes and other kinds of performers in their thirties would be considered in their prime, yet the thirties for dancers often portend retirement.[23] Sometimes even a retirement age in the mid-thirties is generous.

There are exceptions. There are dancers in their fifties and older who demonstrate impressive strength and flexibility (Figs. 8*a–b*). At age sixty-three, award-winning choreographer Gillian Lynne danced on stage for the first time in twenty-five years. There are dancers over forty and fifty who are choreographing, dancing on college stages, performing at Dance Theatre Workshop in New York City. Dancers do not have to be living legends with lots of money and audience goodwill to perform on a stage. Between Maya Plisetskaya and Ruth Page on one end of the age and fame continuum, and the sylphlike teens on the other, I think that some audiences can tolerate a fairly wide range of what they will pay—at least once—to see on stage, in terms of body size and shape and, to a limited extent, weight.

Dancers should carefully consider their options before retiring from dance. In some ways, it is in the dancers' best interests, in terms of physical strength and health, to continue to dance recreationally if not professionally as they age.[24]

Dancers *can* continue to dance in good health much longer (into their forties and beyond) than what is now considered normal (twenties and thirties), and as long as they want. It is not just a matter of being lucky. The question "Does chronological age *invariably* render the dancer artistically and physically dysfunctional?" is to this author—and others—rhetorical. The answer is "Of course not," although the artistic director of either NYCB or ABT and some members of the paying public would probably answer otherwise.

Carmen de Lavallade also says "No," as do Murray Louis, Trisha Brown, Don Redlich, others whose names are less well known, and the people who pay to see them perform. Those named are all modern dancers who are over age fifty and performing. They are, of

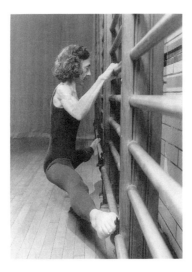

Figure 8a. Kathryn Karipides, age fifty-four, performing her stretch-and-strengthen work at the stall barres in the dance studio at Case Western Reserve University. *(Photo by Mike Sands)*

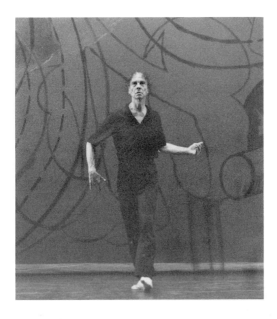

Figure 8b. Merce Cunningham, at age sixty-seven. *(Photo by Jed Downhill)*

course, the exceptions. But their stories (some of which are profiled in this book) tell us that dancers need not be fatalists about their career opportunities in professional dance—even as they age, even as they put on a few more pounds.

It's time for dancers to exercise their rights as well as their bodies. In the abyss of mainstream dance that grooms submissive and obsessive sylphs and Adonises, there may be alternatives. Perhaps older dancers will lead the way in helping others to find the balance in their lives that will allow them to make professional dance their career as well as their passion.

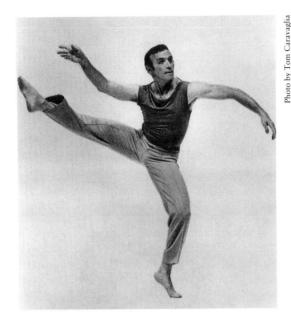

Photo by Tom Caravaglia

Murray Louis

In his mid-sixties Murray Louis is doing it all—dancing, choreograph-ing, co-directing his company, lecturing, writing. For Louis, the overload in his life comes mainly from choreographing: "The creative process is terribly stressful on the inner person, someone upon whom I greatly depend." He has been choreographing for almost forty years and lately he has begun to write about dancers and dance: their audiences, critics, choreography, dance training, teaching, touring, and the financial pressures—subjects that have dominated his life. Louis says:

> The dancer's life is both difficult and painful. One has to find the rewards to compensate for these difficulties. By age twenty-one, a dancer should have a sense of what the reality of this profession is, and by twenty-five or twenty-eight, the initial allure should be based on hard fact. If you stay in this profession, it can prepare you to live your entire life more fully. The whole point of art is that it helps fashion a sanity out of the myriad and random pieces that constitute a lifetime.
>
> For to be an artist-dancer is to penetrate those mysteries

that give you a raison d'être. You must see beyond the immediate pain, the lack of [job] opportunities, inadequate compensation, and often terrible working conditions. This obviously is not a profession for everyone studying dance. But once you are an artist, you remain an artist all your life, and [satisfaction from] your commitment is your reward.

For Louis, there was never any question that dance would be a lifelong career. He knew from the very beginning that stretching his body and mind would not be achieved in three easy lessons. He would say to himself, "This particular stretch is going to take seven months; this will take two years," and set his goals accordingly.

Louis started dancing at age eight or nine. He says, "I was a natural dancer and it all came easily." But it wasn't until he was twenty-two that he began serious artistic training with Alwin Nikolais. It took him seven solid years to retrain his body. Louis reflects on his career in dance:

I completely reoriented my body. Those were very painful years. I was physically numb most of the time. But then at age thirty-two, I really felt I had arrived as an artist. At forty-two, I was doing things I never dreamt were possible. At fifty-two, I gave myself *Déjà-vu,* a witty, charming piece with a sixteen-measure grand plié. I danced this piece all over the world. But then my problems started at fifty-five. My menisci deteriorated. I was ready to have major surgery but Tommy Tune told me about arthroscopy. In eight weeks, I was performing again. Later, the other leg was operated upon, and I continued touring.

I've had some other injuries, all minor but really I'm such an old turtle now. Very little can get to me. I'm just gristle and callouses, but I always move freely and when I land, I never resist the impact. I always go into the movement. I don't grind, I don't lock, I don't resist.

When I warm up, I prepare my body with the intelligence that the Nikolais technique is based upon, and God knows, it works. Today when I choreograph for myself I limit my spectacle air work, and [use] my other skills, such as strength and balance and, of course, my whole range of artistry and quality [of movement].

I dance only one piece on a program today and choreograph more for my company. I don't want to leave this profession crippled and bitter, as is the case with so many of my colleagues. But I must admit I look forward to not having to warm up and maintain my standards of performance someday. I hear there is a life after dancing.

When your audience starts to become uncomfortable watching your physical inabilities, you should not be on stage. I am not dancing the heavy repertory I used to. I am being more selective. Fortunately, I can choreograph for my abilities. I do not want to leave this profession crippled by unlikely challenges. I look forward to choreographic and video projects in the future. [Louis is also a columnist for *Dance Magazine*.]

. . . .

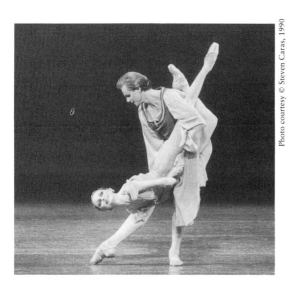

Photo courtesy © Steven Caras, 1990

Patricia McBride

At a gala performance on June 4, 1989, Patricia McBride celebrated thirty years at NYCB. At age forty-six, she was retiring from the company.[25] Francis Mason wrote in a tribute to her:

> She counts eighty-six principal roles. There are probably more. Balanchine made twenty-one for her, and she was resplendent in many he made for others. . . . Patricia McBride has reveled in superb partnerships: Magallanes, Moncion, Villella, d'Amboise, Ludlow, Bonnefoux, Blum, Tomasson, Anderson, Lavery, Lüders, Cook, Baryshnikov, Nureyev, La Fosse, and others. . . . Soubrette, dramatic dancer, and ballerina all in one, McBride has given us the light and the dark, she has given us both the sun and the moon: *Harlequinade* and *La Sonnambula*, *Coppélia* and *In the Night, Who Cares?* and *Dances at a Gathering*, *Tarantella* and *Liebeslieder Waltzer*.[26]

McBride, however, describes herself simply as reliable:

I was always a really hard worker. I remember at one time, in the early 1970s, there was a "ballerina shortage." Melissa Hayden had retired, Gelsey Kirkland had left to join ABT, Violette Verdy and Allegra Kent were both injured and were dancing sporadically. I had to dance most of the repertory, alternating with Kay Mazzo, Karin von Aroldingen, and Sara Leland. It was difficult then. Mr. B. had a single cast for everything. If someone couldn't dance, the ballet would be cancelled. We had to work really hard then.

Today, it's more difficult for the men. For a long time, it's been mostly Sean Lavery, Ib [Anderson], and Adam [Lüders] performing. They have had a hard time, especially with all the lifting.

McBride attributes her longevity to the fact that she has always had to work very hard to keep up. At the School of American Ballet, the entrechats and attitude turns were special challenges. She worked hard to meet them, achieving soloist rank at age seventeen and principal status at age eighteen. She takes great pride in the fact that she has the same joy of dancing as when she started—in part because she has tried to be careful: "I was intelligent. I didn't go for 200-degree extensions."

McBride has retired from NYCB but she hasn't retired from dance. Together with her husband and former NYCB-principal dancer, Jean-Pierre Bonnefoux, she will be performing and teaching to a different audience at Indiana University. It is true that the "Patti McBrides" of the world are few and far between. It is possible, however, for women to dance past the age of forty in ballet, depending on their repertory, their technical training, and the "magicians"—as McBride calls them—and healers they use. Possible, but by no means conventional, at least not yet in the United States.

•   •   •   •   •   •   •   •   •   •   •   •   •   •   •   •   •

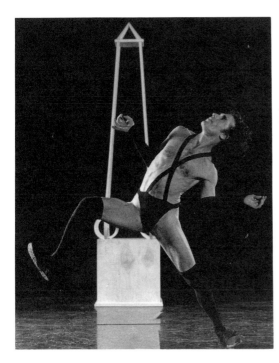

Photo by Cylla von Tiedemann
Courtesy of the Danny Grossman Dance Company

Danny Grossman

As is typical of many independent modern dancers, Danny Grossman dances with, choreographs for, and manages his Toronto-based company. Sometimes it's just too much. The choreography and company promotion, both demanding time and creativity, he finds impossible to time-share. The easy part of his daily work is the dancing, although this wasn't always true.

Grossman danced with the Paul Taylor Dance Company for ten years. In those days of youth, he loved dancing so much that he would have "jumped off a building for it." He not only loved to dance, but also loved to watch dance—the Moiseyev folk dancers, Maya Plisetskaya, Antonio Gades, Alicia Alonso, Donald O'Connor ("all dancers who tore up the floor at parties"). Ethnic influences run strong in his personal life and in his choreography, beginning with his Polish-Hungarian Jewish father and Irish-Catholic mother.

But these inspiring role models weren't enough to carry him through the years of exhausting performances and touring with the Taylor company. After each performance, "everything would hurt." Friends and therapists tried to massage those aches away. Chiropractors and other healers worked on his injured back, calves, and hamstrings on a regular basis, and Don Farnworth, a "physical magician," taught him "to understand (his) own instrument deeply." Probably what saved him more than anything else was leaving the company in 1975 and performing his own choreography.

The first piece he choreographed was a "hang-by-your-neck piece with a ladder," which actually further irritated his neck and lower spine. Since then, he has created more expressive pieces for himself—mature, dramatic roles—that could be performed for twenty years. These aren't run, run, leap roles. These are roles that are difficult to do dramatically and isometrically. In any case, jumps and the leaps really aren't essential to his humorous and humanistic choreographic worldview.

When he does need to use jumps and acrobatic movements in his group works, he has his dancers wear athletic shoes (see Fig. 5). In fact, they usually wear their "best jogging shoes" in most of the dances. This is to protect the dancers—over half of whom are in their mid-thirties and have been with the company for many years—as well as Grossman himself. He still nurses some injuries left over from his Taylor dancing days.

To strengthen his body, he lifts weights and works out with Nautilus machines, and continues to develop the physical and mental technique that has kept him dancing to this day. But it's what he does for his soul—feeding it with as much dance as he can watch—that's most important in keeping him working for himself and for others. Works by Grossman now appear in the repertory of the National Ballet of Canada, Les Grands Ballets Canadiens, the Paris Opéra Ballet, Children's Dance Theatre, Ottowa Ballet, Judith Marcuse Dance Company, and Citidance Company of the City College of New York.

Finding the balance in his life means that he's choreographing a bit less and promoting his company a bit more. In his choreography, quality not quantity is what interests him—and it's what he delivers. In 1988, critic Deidre Kelly commented in the Toronto *Globe and Mail,* "Like Halley's Comet or an eclipse of the sun, a new work by Toronto choreographer Danny Grossman is a rare occurrence that causes witnesses to blink their eyes in wonder. . . . [He is] a strong and dynamic vessel of emotion dancing in the face of the inevitable." Says Grossman, "I feel pulled in many directions, but you can't dance and choreograph and be the artistic director at the same time. You only have energy for one of those jobs each day." Two pieces of choreography a year, some dancing, a lot of artistic management. Now in his late forties, he makes his choices.

. . . .

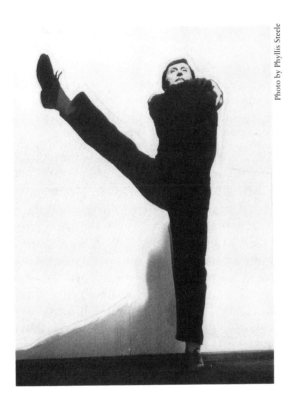

Photo by Phyllis Steele

Daniel Nagrin

Many dance audiences around the country know Daniel Nagrin as a solo performer. He began touring with his solo concerts at the age of forty in 1957. However, he has been a professional dancer since the age of nineteen, and only now is he beginning to write about it.

He has danced in Broadway musicals, Hollywood films, and on television. He has worked with and co-directed a dance company with the legendary Helen Tamiris, choreographed solo concerts that he has toured extensively, and is currently a professor of dance at Arizona State University in Tempe.

In his very cogent writing, he leaves no terpsichorean stone unturned; he has opinions on just about everything to do with staying healthy and dancing. His caveats only serve to lend more authority to his writing:

> This is what I saw/see from where I was/am dancing/living. Not for one moment am I certain of a single statement or thought. I am not yet gone and may not be leaving for a long time, but I am on my way out. For whatever it is worth, it is my obligation to speak now.
>
> It is a vital premise of this book that there are a significant number of choices that are crucial not only to your longevity and your health but to your entire career as an artist. Some of these allow for an infinite number of choices, one of which is not only right for you but is your responsibility to discover for yourself.[27]

His book, *How to Dance Forever: Surviving Against the Odds,* should be read by anyone who's seriously interested in professional dance as a career. His thoughts and reflections on movement mechanics, whether or not they are supported by cited literature, somehow embody what are actually the current state-of-research findings in the respective fields. Quite simply, Nagrin is insightful. He's also a powerful and emotive dancer.

How does one keep dancing past the forty-year barrier? How does one continue to balance the dancing and the choreographing and the touring? How does one keep the passion alive? Read his book.

First, dancers have to manage their days before they can manage their lives: "Rising, we are returning from strange places, known to no other human and barely known to ourselves. . . . I require a minimum of an hour and a half from the moment of waking before I am willing to [dance]. I wake fragile."[28] Nagrin is adamant about daily class (twice a day for a "fully grown student"): "But, then, there are those signals that do say, 'No. Don't dance today.' It may be actual pain, injury, a cold, stomachache, or an inexplicable indisposition."[29]

Although Nagrin is emphatic about the need to dance "full-out" in rehearsal, he is also cautious:

> If your fatigue is such that you fear your coordination is going, speak up. If your choreographer doesn't care or respond to your implicit plea for a break, you have a problem. The world has a problem. There are some terrible people out there, and if it is at all within the range of your power, try to arrange your life so that you work with and for life-enhancing people.[30]

About performance Nagrin writes:

> In Yiddish we would dub a woman or man who risks his/her body in the rigors and glories of dance performance without adequate preparation a "schmuck". . . . What about injury during performance? The show must go on? Impossible to answer. . . . The complexity is complicated by the body's response to injury during performance.[31]

Nagrin refrains from actually advising dancers to continue the performance. Many of the dancers interviewed for this book would stop. As ABT masseur Raymond Serrano warned: "The saying in ballet companies is, 'If you feel it, the injury, when you dance, you're in *big* trouble.' "[32]

After the performance, Nagrin urges the dancer to attend to the body's needs:

> Our vanity thrives on the tangible accolades of devoted fans and unknown members of the audience who feel impelled . . . to come backstage. [But] intensely used muscles must be stretched immediately after use.[33]

And lastly, on sleep, Nagrin writes that "there are no general rules, except two:

1. Find out how much sleep you need.
2. Be a genius and arrange your life so that you get what you need."[34]

Clearly, a particular mind-set is needed for career longevity. Dancers must be active, but not obsessive. It's not how much one trains that's important, it's how one trains.

Two

Injury and Injury Treatment

Dancers sprain ligaments in their back, rupture spinal discs, and tear the cartilage in their knees. They pull the tendons in their shoulders and their groin muscles and strain their calves. In dance, no part of the body is left unscathed, although the lion's share of injuries is found in the lower torso and lower extremities.

Anyone who has ever asked professional dancers about injuries soon learns that their definition of injury is different from that of the average individual. To many dancers, anything short of being sidelined for a week or requiring surgery is hardly an injury.

Dancers interpret the term "injury" in the most practical way: something that prevents them from dancing. It can destroy a career.[1] However, as long as they can perform—strapped, taped, "massaged"/rubbed down, medicated—dancers feel that they're okay. Ask the questions "Are you injured? Have you been injured?" and the answer will probably be no. Ask, "Have you ever danced in pain?" and dancers will smile—of course they have.

Self-Treatment

Table 2 is a list of common dance injuries of the lower body, from the feet up. It is meant to be exemplary, not exhaustive (causes for some of these injuries are listed in Table 1, and the Bibliography includes publications that discuss injuries, treatment, and prevention at greater length). Note also: (1) Not all the treatments listed are considered self-treatment; for example, strapping requires some expertise. (2) There is little mention of heat, here or elsewhere in the chapter. After the initial injury treatment (twenty-four to forty-eight hours, longer in some cases), heat can be very beneficial for symptomatic relief of pain and for facilitating blood flow to the injured area as part of the healing process.[2] (3) Evaluation to determine if faulty technique is a factor of injury causation is vital. Neuromuscular repatterning (see Body Therapies, page 41) or technique modification (see Chapter 3) is recommended for complete rehabilitation. (4) Ice massage and cryotherapy in general are discussed at greater length below. (5) Strengthening regimens and exercises, together with illustrations, are presented in Chapter 5.

Table 2. Injuries and Injury Treatment*

Injury	Treatment
Blisters (assumes area has not become infected; blood blister is not present)	Antiseptic drainage Padding
Plantar Fasciitis (ligament strain causing pain in the arch of the foot and in relevé)	Ice the heel and arch up to 20 minutes at least 3 times a day Aspirin (USE WITH CAUTION) Gentle stretching of the fascia Strapping Heel lifts (ballet orthotic arch support)
"Dancer's Heel" (inflammation of the back of the ankle, the talocalcaneal joint, aggravated by excessive pointe work or structural abnormality—e.g., an extra bone at the back of the ankle, known as the os trigonum)	Ice Aspirin (USE WITH CAUTION) Strapping
Inversion Sprain of the Ankle (injury to outside ankle ligaments)	Elastic bandage (until swelling subsides somewhat) Strapping with pad attached to outer edge of heel (valgus pad) Ice massage Ice therapy/elevation Strengthening

*The information in this table is adapted from Stuart Wright, *Dancer's Guide to Injuries of the Lower Extremity: Diagnosis, Treatment, and Care* (New York: Cornwall Books, 1985) and from L. M. Vincent, *The Dancer's Book of Health* (Pennington, N.J.: Princeton Book Company, Publishers, 1978).

Table 2. Injuries and Injury Treatment (Continued)

Injury	Treatment
Eversion Sprain of the Ankle (less common sprain; injury to the deltoid—inner ankle—ligaments)	See Inversion Sprain treatment Strengthening intrinsic muscles of foot Pad attached to inside of heel (varus pad)
Achilles Tendinitis (one of the most common dance injuries; tendon is chronically overstretched and inflamed, due to fatigue, poor technique)	Ice Aspirin (USE WITH CAUTION) Elevation Heel inserts (at least for street wear) Strapping Stretching Strengthening
Bursitis (inflammation of the bursa between the kneecap and the skin)	Ice Aspirin (USE WITH CAUTION) Compression (elastic wraps or bandages)
Shinsplints (vies with Achilles Tendinitis for most common dance injury; if one wants to become a believer of RICE, try it with shinsplints—this inflammation of the muscle, tendon, or muscle/bone sheath of the lower leg is greatly improved with rest)	Ice Aspirin (USE WITH CAUTION) Heel inserts Padding-strapping Stretching Strengthening
Thigh Strains (hamstrings, quadriceps, adductors)	Ice Compression bandage Strapping Stretching Strengthening

The injuries in Table 2 focus on the lower body. But injuries to the upper torso often result from lifting other dancers, landing from aerial work, and dancing certain modern and jazz choreography. The upper extremities also are not immune from injuries such as shoulder dislocations, elbow tenderness, wrist sprains, and fractures of the metacarpals.[3]

Repeatedly straining muscles and spraining ligaments of the torso result in inflammation that may put pressure on the spinal nerves. Jumping on unresilient floor surfaces can result in compression fractures of the body of the vertebrae. Improper technique in lifting can lead to rupture of the lumbar intervertebral discs. One of the dancers profiled in this book suffers from congenital lower vertebrae problems, yet she continues to work around them.

A common source of pain in the lower back is a weak and tight psoas muscle.[4] The psoas attaches to the lowest thoracic and all of the lumbar vertebrae and inserts on the inside of the femur. The pull on the lower spine is tremendous when that muscle is tight. It invariably is, since we spend most of our lives in hip flexion either as civilians (sitting) or as dancers (in movements requiring the dancer to raise the leg to the front or to bend at the waist).

For all the aforementioned injuries, selective rest of the injured body part is required for healing (but many dancers are unwilling to do that). Also vitally important to the healing process is work on technique, strength, and flexibility.

In terms of self-treatment, however, dancers first need pain relief, from analgesics—aspirin and other anti-inflammatory agents should be used with caution—to strapping or bandaging for support of the injured body part. For injuries to the foot and ankle, some dancers also wear commercial heel inserts or street shoes with heels.

Ice

It may seem banal, but the first line of attack for short-term injury treatment should be the application of ice. Cold minimizes hemorrhaging, although some compression is usually needed to reduce swelling in surrounding tissues (see Figs. 9a–b). As blood flow to the injured site is reduced (vasoconstriction), so is muscle spasm.

Many dancers do not ice their injuries. Certainly, when performing or rehearsing it's difficult.

Applying ice requires motivation; it takes time. Some injuries (lower back, groin) are difficult to ice. There are dancers who believe that their injuries are "too deep" to ice. When dancers see others with ice packs, the immediate question is "What happened to you?" They expect some acute injury to be responsible. Tendinitis and bursitis respond very well to cold application, so that dancers should not feel that they're "wasting time" if they take time to apply ice to a chronic injury.

Ice can be systematically applied (cryotherapy) to injured tissue by using ice packs (a bag of crushed ice or refreezable gel packs) for no more than twenty to thirty minutes at a time, ice baths for even less

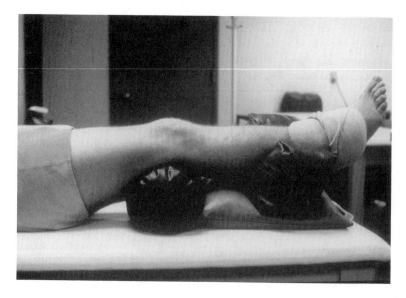

Figure 9a. A lateral ankle sprain is treated with ICE (Ice-Compression-Elevation). The crushed ice is held on the ankle with an elastic wrap. Some compression is needed to minimize swelling in and about other tissues. *(Photo by Carol Teitz, M.D.)*

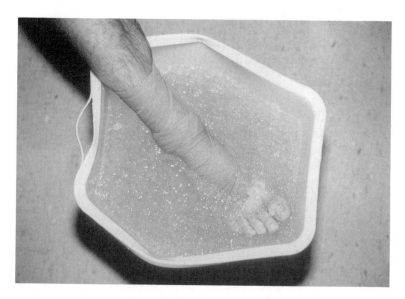

Figure 9b. Ice bath. After the ice bath, the bandage can be removed and a dry wrap applied. The foot may be placed in the ice bath without wrapping as long as it is moved around. *(Photo by Carol Teitz, M.D.)*

time, or ice massage, assuming there are no neurovascular or circulatory contraindications. For ice massage, one can freeze water in a disposable cup and then peel or cut away the top of the cup, which easily allows the ice to come into contact with the skin. Companies and schools should keep ice trays and disposable cups filled.

The benefits of cryotherapy are widely recognized. In general, it is accepted as safe and there are few medical complications resulting from it. The ice should be repositioned occasionally, checking carefully to ensure that it is not damaging superficial tissues (i.e., causing an ice burn).[5]

Critical to the healing process is maintaining the mobility of the joint. This is especially true at the "remodeling" stage of injury-healing. As an initial response to healing, certain vascular changes (e.g., white blood cells removing dead tissue at the site of injury) result in swelling and redness. After twenty-four to forty-eight hours, the body begins to replace the injured tissue with strands of the protein, collagen.

If the joint is not allowed to be mobile, the collagen will grow into scar tissue that is weaker and more inelastic than the original tendon structure. Eventually, adhesions are produced. These are wisplike protrusions from the sheath covering the tendon. They restrict the mobility of the joint, making the area more susceptible to reinjury. The analgesic effect of ice can allow the joint to remain relatively mobile, thus helping to prevent the formation of scar tissue and adhesions.

Medics and Other Healers

The degree to which an injury affects the performing ability of a dancer depends on the severity and frequency of the injury, the repertory that is being danced, and the treatment that is prescribed and followed. Self-treatment makes sense only when the causal factors of injury have been identified and medical intervention is not indicated.

The process of identifying the causal factors of injury should be part of a diagnosis by a healthcare professional. There are any number of types of "healers" that may be involved in a dancer's physical evaluation and rehabilitation. Table 3 is a list of common, mostly Western-oriented "healers" who treat dance injuries. Some normative degrees or qualifications are given. Daniel Nagrin's *How*

Table 3. Examples of Healers for Treatment of Dance Injuries

Acupuncturist (certified, licensed)
Athletic Trainer (M.S., M.S.P.E.)
Body/Movement Therapist* (D.T.R., C.M.A.; certified, licensed)
Chiropractor (D.C.)
Dietician (R.D.)
Kinesiologist (M.S. and/or Ph.D.)
Healers (spiritual, e.g., laying on of hands)
Homeopath (certified, licensed)
Massage Therapist (certified, licensed)
Nutritionist (M.S. and/or Ph.D.)
Osteopathic Physician (D.O.)
Physical Therapist (P.T., M.S., M.P.T.)
Physicians and Surgeons (M.D.):
    General practitioner; Internist; Orthopedist; Radiologist; Neurologist;
    Psychiatrist
Podiatrist (D.P.M.)
Psychotherapist (L.C.S.W., M.F.C.T., Ph.D.)
Rolfing Practitioner (certified, licensed)
Shiatsu Practitioner (certified, licensed)
Specialists (e.g., Pilates; certified, licensed)

---

*Body/movement therapists practice any one of a number of body therapies (Alexander, Bartenieff Fundamentals, Feldenkrais, Ideokinesis). Practitioners of Body-Mind Centering who have worked with Bonnie Bainbridge-Cohen can also be included. None of them need to be Certified Movement Analysts (C.M.A.s), but most C.M.A.s are well versed in at least Bartenieff Fundamentals.

to Dance Forever: Surviving Against the Odds (pp. 119–166) offers an excellent description of some of these "healers" and their methods of treatment.

The objective of any treatment program must surely be to return the dancer to the same, if not greater, preinjury physical and functional condition. How this is achieved depends on a variety of factors, not the least of which are money and the diversity of available "healers" and facilities that dancers can trust.

Of all the types of "healers" listed in Table 3, massage therapists, physical therapists, and chiropractors are often the top choices for dancers. Daniel Nagrin provides a very thoughtful discussion on the restorative nature of touch therapies in general.[6] He argues that the mere act of touching is healing, fulfilling a basic human need for attention and care, especially when tissue is injured.

Massage may be popular among dancers, but the other healing options should not be discounted.[7] For example, psychotherapy is also popular in helping dancers deal with the stresses of their career, especially when such service is covered by a health insurance plan.

Physical therapy may also be part of a total rehabilitation program. The body therapies are generally regarded as critical for learning correct technique and movement repatterning.

Massage

Many dancers enjoy massage, not so much for injury treatment as for relaxation and general healing (Fig. 10). Massage is actually a fairly broad category. Certainly in licensing masseurs and masseuses there is a wide range in the number of hours required to complete a course of instruction. Some dancers prefer to call their massage treatments deep frictioning work, structural integration, or body sculpturing. A few professional companies have massage practitioners on staff.

A case in point is ABT. Raymond Serrano has been with the company for sixteen years; for the past three years, he has been the company's resident and touring massage practitioner. Just now weaning himself from character roles, he still joins company members in class and rehearsal. He says that he does a lot of work on the female

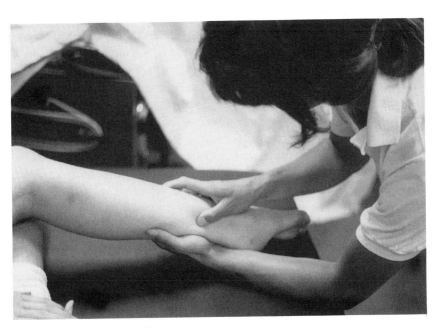

Figure 10. Massage therapy. Massage is an example of a "touch therapy" used to mobilize scar tissue and increase blood circulation to an injured area. Massage may also include relaxation therapies, such as therapeutic laying on of hands, stretch and release exercises, and breathing sequences. *(Photo by Richard Braver, D.P.M.)*

dancers' bruised and swollen feet "to help move the fluid out of the foot."[8]

Serrano varies how deeply he manipulates the soft tissues, depending how far dancers are in a rehabilitation program. He is quick to note that massage is used for short-term needs as well as long-term recovery. Also, it is easily abused: "Sometimes you get an eleventh-hour appeal. . . . I do whatever I can . . . to enhance the dancers' performance in helping them keep from getting injured. . . . They don't like it because it *hurts*, but they let me do it because it *works*."

Massage can mobilize tissue by breaking down adhesions and scar tissue and increasing blood circulation. However, a problem with massage is that tissue can become easily irritated in the hands of a practitioner keen on "going deep," but not familiar with primary and secondary structures that may be irritated in the process. Dancers also complain about the expense of massage, quoting fees of thirty-five to seventy-five dollars per hour.

Physical Therapy

In a conventional rehabilitative program, the physician, podiatrist, or osteopathic physician may prescribe the general course of treatment, but it is the physical therapist who develops and administers it.

Professionals trained in physical therapy are usually able to offer conditioning as well as therapeutic programs. Furthermore, if therapists have considerable clinical experience working with dancers, they will also be able to address the faulty technique that is causing the injury to occur and recur.

There is no doubt that physical therapy requires a time commitment of the injured dancer. It is not atypical for a patient to need three visits a week for six weeks to three months. If the physical therapist is not associated with a dance company and located close to its studios, appointments for company dancers can be a scheduling nightmare. This is because physical therapists are very busy, especially the ones with dance-related clinical experience—and these are the ones that dancers should try to choose (see the Directory of Selected Dance/Arts Medicine Clinics; many have associated physical therapists).

Physical therapy may also be a financial drain if the dancer's private or company insurance does not cover physical therapy. Some clinics and practices offer such service for dance students and professionals on a sliding scale. Sometimes, coverage may be provided in a Health Maintenance Organization (HMO) plan, but the HMO may require that the patient pass a number of barriers (i.e., visits first to a general practitioner and then an orthopedist) before being awarded physical therapy services. Don't lose heart: the more patients who force the issue, the easier it will become for other HMO participants.

Physical therapy makes use of many different modalities. These include hot packs, cold packs, deep-tissue massage, ultrasound, whirlpool, connective tissue mobilization, joint mobilization, spinal mobilization, "spray and stretch," and electrical stimulation. For the most part, they are physically gratifying. Whether they actually help to rehabilitate and discharge the patient—completely cured and ready to embark on a self-healing regimen—is something else. But that, ostensibly, is the goal.

Once dancers see the benefits of physical therapy, they may push their activity for a week or longer, knowing that the physical therapist will always be there (financial constraints notwithstanding) to mobilize the painfully tight and weak tendons and ligaments they overuse. Then they'll have a little relief, in time for the next rehearsal and performance push.

One kinesiologist I spoke to pushes her dancing to the limit—forcing turnout at the hips and knees, overstretching the arches in her foot. She sometimes uses her foot as a lever against heavy furniture for resistance. But no matter. In her physical therapy practice she has unlimited equipment with which to treat the incessant injuries. This is an extreme example of abuse of physical therapy services.

Body Therapies

The body therapy innovators have explored the relationship between the mind and body—between imaging movement and effecting it. As such, the body therapies, or rather the men and women who have pioneered them, have given dancers a new vision of human movement—for retraining and reeducating the body, for rehabilitating it from injury, and for enhancing the quality of performance.

The body therapies are really an amalgam of movement education styles and philosophies based in gymnastics, neurology, physiological psychology, Eastern philosophies, principles of Delsarte and Dalcroze, and even the martial arts. Almost all focus on poor muscular habits in technique and training or early developmental patterns of mobility that predispose the dancer to injury.

The body therapies help dancers to identify areas of neuromuscular tenseness and inefficient movement patterns and to be spatially aware of body parts. This enables them to sense when the head is too far forward of the body, the shoulders lifted, the lower back arched. One has to recognize the locus of tension—the source of poor movement habits—before there can be any correction or adjustment. Otherwise, the new habit superimposed over the old will create further distortions and harmful movement patterns.

Almost all the body therapies emphasize movement patterns rather than individual movements. Muscular action does not occur in isolation. Groups of muscles are involved and different parts of the same muscles are often responsible for different actions, some of which are only evident through electromyographic recordings of the contractile components of the muscle fibers. Thus, it is often difficult to correct a complex movement once it is initiated. Where does the student begin? The following discussion presents four of the more common body therapies. For others, see the Bibliography.

BARTENIEFF FUNDAMENTALS

Inefficient movement patterns can lead to injury through muscle misuse or overuse, resulting in muscle imbalance and fatigue. In order to break this cycle, the inefficient pattern must be identified and a more functional movement pattern developed.

The Fundamentals, a series of movement sequences developed by Irmgard Bartenieff, allows for a systematic investigation of such muscle use and movement patterns (these sequences are now an integral part of the Laban Movement Analysis system in the United States).

In *Body Movement: Coping with the Environment,*[9] Bartenieff presents some basic movement sequences that emphasize the diagonal connections between lower and upper extremities and the changing shape of the whole spine from the base of the skull to the coccyx. An example is the thigh lift:

> *Thigh lift* ("femoral flexion"), pre-lift. The objective of the thigh lift is to use primarily the iliopsoas muscle to isolate hip flexion. Lying in a supine position with the arms to the side and palms on the floor, the abdomen hollows and one foot slides toward the ischium upon exhalation, the knee bending. The student is asked

to feel the continuous folding of the inguinal or groin area and at the same time feel the lengthening of the lower back along the floor. In addition, there is a head-tail, heel-coccyx connection that must be maintained. Returning to the start position requires that the movement be initiated with the hip, not the knee.

Thigh lift, lift. The initiation of the femoral flexion is the same, but a graded pelvic tilt might be added. The thigh moves toward the chest upon exhalation—the student is asked to think about the foot moving rather than the upper thigh. The weight of the upper body is cradled by the scapula. As with all the movement sequences, the student is encouraged to think of the quality of the movement. Pushing, pulling, or any movements with unnecessary tension are discouraged.

Other Fundamentals sequences used to evaluate movement patterns include the pelvic forward (sagittal) shift, the pelvic lateral shift, folding and unfolding of alternate sides of the body (body-half relationship), relaxing the lower torso side-to-side (knee lowering or "drop"), arm circles, a diagonal sit-up (that develops into full-body spiraling patterns), and others. In each sequence, Bartenieff has given its purpose and function, instructions for performing the action, notes on what the student should be feeling and should avoid, and the pedestrian functions for which the movement is used.

With each movement sequence, it is important to find its correct initiation. This means that the student must find the part of the body in which a particular movement begins to coordinate the desired movement sequence. As Martha Myers and Marian Horosko point out, "If the first step in the sequence is wrong, the whole neuromuscular 'event' is doomed."[10]

One way to determine the specific point of initiation for a complex movement pattern is to understand the requisite dynamic alignment—the neuromuscular patterning that responds accurately and sensitively to changes in standing, walking, and sitting. Myers has developed an exercise sequence that trains dancers in dynamic alignment: she uses touch, breath, and imaged movement to help them activate abdominal, hip, and pelvic musculature from the Moslem-prayer position (kneeling, buttocks resting on heels, torso rounded forward).

In sum, training in Bartenieff Fundamentals allows for screening for injury potential, evaluation of technique in terms of efficiency of movement and potential for injury, and rehabilitating the dancer in more efficient movement patterns. Rather than being an end in itself, it allows the student to meet the demands of advanced work in dance.[11]

IDEOKINESIS

According to Lulu Sweigard, the initiation and inhibition of impulses to specific muscles is made possible by visualizing particular movement patterns. This visualization is referred to as "ideokinesis"—the conceptualization of movement with the purpose of promoting a balanced skeletal alignment and greater efficiency in movement. As is clear from Sweigard's book, *Human Movement Potential: Its Ideokinetic Facilitation*,[12] ideokinesis is both science and art.

In her book, Sweigard talks about using the imagination to work on correct alignment. Such change is subcortically controlled. This requires that students concentrate on envisioning movement occurring within their body (e.g., in a "perfect" plié), without contributing any physical effort to its performance.

Sweigard also discusses at some length the *teaching* of visualization technique. There are some important prerequisites teachers must have before they are competent to guide their students ideokinetically to better musculoskeletal balance: a concept of good skeletal alignment based on anatomy and biomechanics, knowledge of typical faulty alignment, the ability to determine where and in what direction movement is needed to bring the skeleton into correct alignment, and the ability to note alignment problems in the habitual movement patterns of students.

Above all, the teacher must be able to design images to which the student can relate. In Chapters 20 and 21 of *Human Movement Potential,* Sweigard gives guidelines, such as:

1. Each imagined movement must make sense in terms of what is possible with the usual skeletal structure.
2. Movement should be described in terms of images and experiences that are familiar to the students.
3. Many different images for each line-of-movement should be designed so as to avoid repetition.

How should the movement be presented? Again, Sweigard presents guidelines. The purpose of the imagined movement must be clearly stated, graphically described, and specific—perhaps using a skeleton for illustration. The image must also be developed with words, such as *imagine, visualize, as if, watch,* and *pretend.* The following are some examples of Sweigard's visualizations:

> In the constructive rest position (a position used for reducing muscle strain and balancing the muscles before imaging movement): the image of the "empty suit" is used for locating and directing imagined movement in the body—the trousers are supported at the knees by the cross-bar of an imaginary hanger extended from the ceiling; the arms of the coat rest across the chest and front of the coat. The suit is disheveled. Movements are then prescribed to straighten out the suit such as "Watch the upper part (thigh) of the trouser leg collapsing together as its knee is supported over the cross-bar of the hanger."[13]
>
> To lengthen the spine downward: this image begins with the instructions, "Visualize the buttocks as unbaked loaves of dough and watch them slide downward to the back of the heels."[14]
>
> To widen across the back of the pelvis: this image begins with the instructions, "Imagine the pelvis as a toy accordion with handles on either side and vertical pleats on the front and back. Watch the accordion being opened wide in back to remove all pleats."[15] ". . . Watch hip pockets on the back of the pelvis moving around to the front."[16]

Sweigard's work is rich with images for movement awareness and correction. In addition, she discusses a variety of techniques to reduce strain and improve neuromuscular coordination in daily movements. Irene Dowd,[17] building on Sweigard's work, offers imagery for even more complex dance movement, such as an arabesque. She, too, encourages students to imagine—with eyes in each vertebra and skin cells of the back that are opening to look into a huge mirror. She asks students to imagine, not to feel (this comes later) the movement, to visualize that the arabesque is supported from behind the body.

Ideokinesis offers enormous possibilities for developing more efficient movement mechanics. Self-correction is possible after considerable self-education.

ALEXANDER TECHNIQUE

As in ideokinesis, the concept of "inhibition" is also important in the Alexander technique. It is believed that once students are aware of inefficient movement patterns (e.g., "locking" the knees in relevé position) they can learn to inhibit them, replacing them with more functional movement adjustments. This requires what Alexander termed "conscious control."

The technique was developed by F. Matthias Alexander as a way of improving "the use of the self." Developed originally for actors, it has been a part of the program at the Theatre Center of the Juilliard School since its opening in 1968. It is interesting to note that Alexander's observations and experiments on vocal problems have been applauded by noted scientists such as ethologist Nikolaas Tinbergen.

Alexander hypothesized that in each of us there is an "integrating mechanism" that would produce better coordination and functioning if allowed to operate without interference. This mechanism he called "primary control": "I discovered that a certain use of the head in relation to the neck, and of the head and neck in relation to the torso and other parts of the organism . . . constituted a primary control of the organism *as a whole.*"[18] Thus the term refers to a head balanced freely and easily on the end of the spine. This is achieved by thinking of the head "forward and up," activating the erector muscles along the length of the spine. In this technique, emphasis is put on the upper torso—in particular the cervical spine—rather than, for example, the inner shaping of the torso as in Bartenieff Fundamentals.

The teachers assist students through hands-on work and verbal cues to activate their primary control. The technique is traditionally taught one-on-one, since touch is such an important part of the directing or "conscious control" that the teacher provides. (Teachers of the technique must learn to communicate with their hands, as Alexander did.) Eventually, the student is able to activate the conscious control without any direction from a teacher.[19]

A typical Alexander lesson might be the following:

> The student may be lying on a table that is slightly higher and wider than a massage table. The teacher gently talks to and touches the student. The teacher repeatedly returns to the head and neck, "because it is the relationship of the head, neck and spine that governs his primary control." In addition, the teacher will also work with the student in activities that involve the use of a chair. Through verbal and tactile cues, the teacher helps the

student to sit and stand. As the student becomes more familiar with the technique, the teacher will give primarily verbal cues during the instruction.[20]

It is the job of the Alexander teacher to help the student discover efficient, tension-free movement patterns; preferably individually, but when necessary, in groups (as is the case at the American Dance Festival, where the Alexander technique has been taught in groups for over ten years). Martha Myers notes that the change in students' movement has been dramatic:

> [The students] become more aware of themselves and of others around them, and this learning feeds directly into technique, improvisation, and composition classes. Students who've studied Alexander technique find it easier to be placed up and over the legs rather than behind, resting backwards, a common problem among late-starting students. Their head usage, particularly in spotting, improves dramatically, and the improved coordination reverberates down the spine and into other movements, especially turns.[21]

Myers also believes that since the major sensory organs are located in the head, changing the orientation of the head and neck can alter perceptions of oneself and one's environment. It is a welcome change. Once students become familiar with the technique and recognize that this is indeed the "real stuff" (i.e., real technical training), they find their discoveries exhilarating.

Myers warns that dancers must take risks and let go of what they think is "right" and "correct" before they can learn more efficient ways of moving. She adds, "In the process, they make 'mistakes.' The more in tune with their bodies they become, however, the more able they are to go beyond accustomed boundaries, still maintaining the body's integrity to avoid injury."[22]

FELDENKRAIS

Moshe Feldenkrais's approach to body reeducation also emphasizes finding correct alignment and examining movement patterns carefully. Feldenkrais emphasizes early developmental patterns of human mobility and "organic" (deep) breathing patterns. He believes that the correction of movement is the best means of self-improvement.

In his book, *Awareness Through Movement*,[23] he presents twelve lessons from more than 1,000 given at the Feldenkrais Institute. He advises that students should perform one lesson every evening before going to sleep, repeating each movement ten times and increasing progressively to twenty-five. In time, it is possible to repeat a movement perhaps 100 times, both slowly and quickly (not hurried). To do the exercises, choose an area of the floor large enough to allow the body to extend in all directions. A thick mat may be used.

Lesson 1 discusses "What is good posture?" It involves sitting on the front edge of a chair and letting the body rock forward and backward in movements that eventually become larger. Feldenkrais argues that no effort greater than that involved in the rocking movement is required to get up. How is this possible? Some pointers:

> Avoid conscious mobilization of the leg muscles (on the swing forward, think about lifting the knees and feet from the floor, rather than lifting the thighs). Feel whether or not the neck muscles are tensed or relaxed by pulling the hair at the top of the head gently in line with the cervical spine.[24]

In Lesson 2, Feldenkrais teaches students to use specific large muscle groups for heavy work. Lesson 3 gives specific exercises to scan the state of the body. Most of these ask students to lie on the floor on their stomachs, paying attention to the manner in which the body parts make contact with the floor. Movements such as raising the arm until the back of the hand is off the floor are repeated. The movements build upon themselves—lifting the elbow, followed by the whole arm, the shoulders, the legs, then alternately raising arm and leg. Lesson 4 concentrates on breathing patterns used in conjunction with seesaw movements of the body—on the side, on the back, and while kneeling.

Lesson 5 coordinates the flexor and extensor muscles with twisting or rocking movements; Lesson 6 shows differentiation of pelvic movements with rotation of the pelvis; and Lesson 7 focuses on the carriage of the head, again with twisting movements of the upper body in opposition to the lower (and thus effectively using the deeper abdominal muscles: the internal and external obliques). Lesson 8, "Perfecting the Self-image," contains exercises in a sitting position and exercises that require rolling from sitting to lying positions and back to sitting.

Lesson 9 looks at spatial relationships, particularly in the face (moving the nose, focusing attention on the ear lobe, and so on). Lesson 10 emphasizes the movement of the eyes, which he believes coordinates the body movements and is linked to the movement of the neck muscles. Lesson 11 suggests techniques for "completion of the self-image" by comparing the sensation in parts of the body of which one is conscious with those parts of which one is not. Finally, Lesson 12 presents guidelines for visualizing the movements of the lung, such as stretching, spreading, and pulling.

Feldenkrais writes about increasing the student's sensibilities— the ability to feel and visualize—as the only way to redirect the force of habit. If indeed awareness is the highest stage in human development, then improvement of body and movement awareness is critical to freeing students' energies for creative work. Feldenkrais, and his certified movement instructors, are helping to spread that message.[25]

Body Therapies and Professional Dancers

In order for dancers to understand a body therapy, they must take time to adjust the sequence of movements they habitually perform. Then, they must be willing to spend more time realigning the body, imaging movement, and working on coordination patterns.[26] For some this is possible only through studying body therapies; others may find the correction through technique class or physical therapy. Still others are quick to acknowledge that it is not an either/or situation—the body therapies can easily be incorporated into other training regimens.

The older dancers whom I interviewed for this book, however, seem to be sharply divided on the efficacy of the body therapies. Murray Louis contends:

> I feel if you must go to other systems for corrective methods, the dance technique you have been studying has in a sense shortchanged you, and there are many dance techniques taught which are very limited in their scope. . . . There are processes to help speed certain development. These, I think, are useful, but on the whole I feel dancers who seek out these practices are indulging themselves and enjoying the sensual pleasures of one-on-one manipulation.

Among the dancers who used the body therapies, Alexander technique seemed to be the most popular. Danny Grossman said that the work he does is "like Alexander;" it is this "like Alexander" work that kept him dancing for Paul Taylor for ten years without missing one performance, using the work for injury treatment as well as injury prevention.

The dancers who practiced body therapies were very devoted to them, either to one in particular or to several; a dancer at NYCB had worked with Moshe Feldenkrais in Israel and so preferred that technique. Kelly Holt stated, "I have tried many of the body therapies—too numerous to mention. I do not have a manic dedication to correction but more one of inquiry—what more can I find out?"

What does one conclude from all this? Depending on the practitioner with whom one works, the body therapies can be enormously helpful—even for virtuoso dancers. Lessons may be expensive, but group sessions can be arranged so that costs are divided among the participants. For dancers who are ready to break harmful movement patterns and let go of inappropriate solutions to dance movement problems, the lessons are well worth the investment. Injured dancers, who are beginning a process of reeducation and training to prevent further trauma to connective tissue, will especially find the body therapies useful.

Rehabilitation

In general, a total rehabilitation program conventionally consists of three steps.

1. Evaluation by a Licensed M.D. and Physical Therapist of the Dancer's Health, Technique, and Working Environment. This evaluation may be cursory. The physician may decide that more time is needed before an accurate diagnosis can be made or that diagnostic tests, such as a bone scan, are needed. Otherwise, it is at this point that the course of treatment—aggressive/invasive or conservative— will be prescribed. Aggressive treatment might involve in- or out-patient surgery, while conservative treatment will probably include physical therapy. If an aggressive course of treatment is recommended or if the injury is debilitating, a second opinion is usually warranted.

2. Sessions of Therapeutic and Rehabilitative Work. These may include physical therapy, massage, body therapies, acupuncture, Rolfing, Shiatsu, and others. Note that these treatments are not mutually exclusive; for example, massage can be included as a component of physical therapy. Short-term treatments such as prescription medications, structural devices (braces, supports), and even cortisone or enzyme injections (which may have serious long-term effects) may only treat the symptoms while causal factors of injury and pain are not addressed.

3. STRENGTHENING AND FLEXIBILITY EXERCISES. As part of the re-habilitative program, general conditioning and fitness work and counseling regarding injury prevention may also be given. Such counseling might include changes in technique, diet, and training schedules. Examples of rehabilitation using the three steps are given below.

Rehabilitation is not a "quick-fix" so that the dancer can immediately return to performing. Rather, the dancer is taught that rehabilitation is a continuous process. It is an act of taking control of one's life, of taking the time to heal and condition the body. Allan Ryan and Robert Stephens note that "every step in the process is part of a coordinated chain which is connected with the succeeding steps to reach the desired goal. As far as the dancer is concerned it is an active rather than a passive process."[27]

Sample Rehabilitation Program: Ankle Tendinitis

1. EVALUATION. Tendinitis around the ankle joint can be either acute—resulting from accidental injury to the ankle—or chronic.[28] In chronic tendinitis, the injury is recurring. Improper dance technique is usually a major contributing factor to the injury. Problems with technique include excessive rolling in (eversion, "winging") or rolling out (inversion, "sickling") of the foot (discussed at length in Chapter 3).

In addition to improper dance technique, anatomical limitations, such as a high instep, and poor strength or flexibility of affected muscles and tendons also cause injury. In addition to recommending a course of physical therapy and conditioning, the evaluation may also indicate the need for corrective devices or "orthotics." Dr. Richard Braver has developed one for dancers that slips onto the bottom of the dancer's foot (Fig. 11).

Although not aesthetically pleasing, the orthotic is at least functional during class and rehearsal, and some dancers also use it in performance. It should not be regarded as a substitute for the strengthening and flexibility work that is necessary to correct alignment and muscle use. It is most useful for structural (anatomical) corrections.

2. THERAPEUTIC MODALITIES AND PROCEDURES. The physical therapist usually follows a physician's prescription for which treatment modalities should be used. For tendinitis in the ankle joint, these

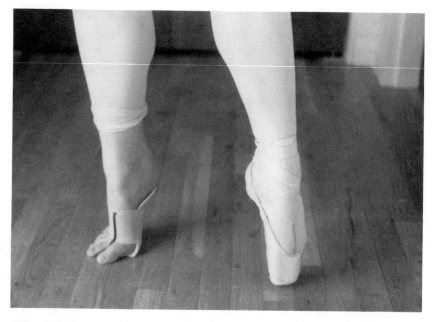

Figure 11. An orthotic limits excessive rolling in and rolling out of the foot and repositions joints to alleviate pressure put on muscles and tendons. *(Photo by Richard Braver, D.P.M.)*

might include ice/cold packs, massage, ultrasound, and connective tissue mobilization.[29]

3. STRENGTHENING AND FLEXIBILITY EXERCISES needed to correct poor alignment and muscle imbalances. For ankle tendinitis, the course of strengthening and flexibility work is clear. Dancers, especially in ballet, spend much of their life perfecting their hip turnout. This means that the outward hip and thigh muscles are constantly used and perhaps strengthened while the inner thigh muscles are usually stretched. This imbalance is obvious when a dancer is spotted walking down the street "toed-out." It predisposes the dancer to tendinitis in the ankle joint, since the inside of the ankle is constantly "on stretch." To correct this imbalance, dancers have to strengthen the inside thighs and stretch the stronger outer hip, thigh, and buttocks muscles.

Dancers work their Achilles tendons with every extension or pointing of the feet. Consequently, the tendon-muscle structure on the back of the legs is tight and requires concerted stretching. Likewise, the muscles along the front of the leg and ankle are constantly strained in an attempt to counterbalance the pull of the Achilles along the back of the heel. The muscles in the front of the leg must be strengthened (exercises for this are illustrated in Chapter 4; an exercise that also increases muscular endurance along the front of the leg can be done standing or in a deep lunge position, without using a band: tap the foot, heel planted firmly on the ground and the foot flexing maximally to the point of reasonable discomfort.)

Sample Rehabilitation Program: Shoulder Impingement

1. EVALUATION. At ABT, among principal male dancers shoulder impingement syndrome is a common problem. It is an overuse injury caused in part by excessive lifting, especially in overhead lifts, and in part by structural conditions (such as an anatomically narrow space in which the head of the humerus moves relative to the acromion process and the lateral aspect of the clavicle).[30] Weak deltoid muscles and excessive scar tissue contribute to this characteristically painful syndrome. A full evaluation by a healthcare professional at the time of injury is essential for rehabilitation.

2. THERAPEUTIC MODALITIES AND PROCEDURES. Methods of rehabilitation for this condition will differ, depending on the severity of the injury. Besides application of cold and rest from lifting activities, treatment may include gentle soft tissue mobilization in the shoulder joint, manipulation/lengthening of tight shoulder-girdle muscles, electrical stimulation, or deep friction massage.

In addition, artificial bracing high on the arm directly over the biceps tendon may be used. If aspirin and other anti-inflammatories are administered, they must be monitored closely for side effects. Cortisone injections may also be prescribed, although they are less popular now than in the past; if given frequently or without caution, they increase the risk of tendon rupture.

3. STRENGTHENING AND FLEXIBILITY EXERCISES. These include stretching and strengthening of the muscles that comprise the rotator cuff (Figs. 12a–e). Stretching is usually initiated immediately, and then strengthening when some healing has occurred. Strengthening exercises focused on the rotator muscles below the level of impingement are helpful. Surgical tubing, rubber bands, and light free weights may also be used.[31]

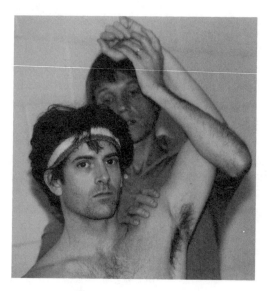

Figure 12a. Peter Marshall, company physical therapist, working with principal dancer Victor Barbee. Physical therapy involves evaluating the extent of injury as well as the general condition of the musculature. *(Photos by Megan Lawrence)*

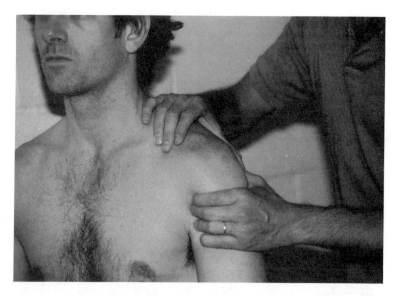

Figure 12b. Shoulder mobilization: Posterior glide of the humerus.

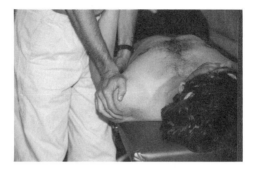

Figure 12c. Shoulder mobilization: Anterior glide of the humerus.

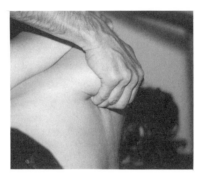

Figure 12d. Deep-tissue mobilization to "release" the subscapularis muscle.

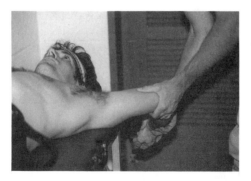

Figure 12e. Stretching the inward rotators of the shoulder joint, in particular, the latissimus dorsi.

Sample Rehabilitation Program: Posterior Compression of the Lower Lumbar Spine

1. EVALUATION. Repetitive lumbar compression is the result of lifting and jumping, which strain the lumbar musculature. Musculoskeletal imbalance is the most significant factor that predisposes dancers to develop compressive or excessive strain syndrome. The imbalance most often involves a tight psoas muscle and weak abdominal and paravertebral musculature. Overload in training, environmental factors such as unresilient floors or tight costumes, lifting a partner mismatched in height or weight or with improper timing, may also be to blame (these factors are treated in Chapters 3 and 4).[32]

2. THERAPEUTIC MODALITIES AND PROCEDURES. Initial treatment consists of massage, electrical stimulation, and ice. Manual mobilization of the lower-thoracic/upper-lumbar spine, shoulder-girdle stretching, and hip stretching assisted by a physical therapist are recommended.

3. STRENGTHENING AND FLEXIBILITY EXERCISES. More than a rehabilitative program, the Group Back Education Program at NYCB, developed and coordinated by physical therapist Elizabeth Henry, has as its main goal injury prevention. The exercises are performed in three sets of ten repetitions and include lumbar bracing and stabilization.

In "bracing," a neutral spine position is assumed, then the muscles of the side, stomach, and back are contracted. In the neutral spine position, a vertical compression force applied through the shoulders should not reveal any evidence of strain of the lumbar structures. The spine is neither excessively stiff nor straight. Rather, the feeling should be of "support," with the navel pressed toward the spine, not to flatten the lumbar curve, but to fully engage the abdominal muscles. It is these muscles that will assist in supporting the lower spine during lifting and jumping movements.

The exercise can be made more difficult by adding marching movements of the legs (Fig. 13) or arms. Dynamic stabilization of the spine for various barre exercises is also emphasized.

Stretching exercises include those for tight hip flexors. Hip flexors must be stretched to allow production of normal range of motion at the hip joint (an example of this type of stretch is seen in Figure 29).

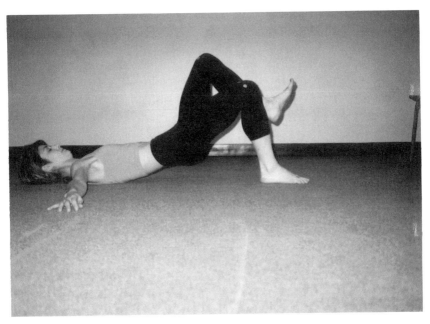

Figure 13. Barbara Gagas demonstrates abdominal bracing exercise. *(Photo by Marika Molnar, P.T.)*

Injury Prevention

Worse perhaps than being injured in dance is the *fear* of injury, of debilitating pain, of capricious muscle spasms, of career setback. After a serious injury, dancers are motivated to learn why and how they were injured. They become more sensitive to the warning signs of the pain. They know when they are being destructive of their bodies.

When company directors jokingly inform their dancers that "if you rip the muscles, they grow back longer," dancers know they're in big trouble if they don't look out for themselves. They have to take responsibility for treating their injuries, conditioning their bodies, and preventing further injury: no one else will.

What are the important causes of injury? The list is endless—the stressful and competitive nature of professional dance, faulty technique, inefficient movement mechanics, inadequate warm-up, insufficient flexibility, poor preseason muscle strength, poor cardio-vascular and muscular endurance, muscle imbalances, scheduling of rehearsals and performance, changes in intensity of dance training or performance, anatomical limitations, biomechanical factors, hard floors, cold theatres, fatigue, poor nutrition.

Many of these causes can be distilled into two major problem areas. The first is poor technique (see Chapter 3). No one has a perfect line. Whether or not a dancer has anatomical abnormalities, few have over 70 degrees of external hip rotation in shooting for the ideal of 90 degrees. The bottom line is technical correction, the best way to prevent injuries. That means that muscles must be sufficiently strong and flexible and neuromuscular patterning adequately developed to allow for proper and safe execution of technically correct movement (see Chapter 4).

The second problem area comprises environmental, administrative, and artistic factors, over which dancers have little control—flooring, restrictive costumes, exhausting touring schedules, pathogenic choreography (see Chapters 1 and 6). What does that leave? Warm-up.

Warming Up

Some dancers like to warm up. Some dancers love to warm up. Others consider it drudgery—a routine they must or should perform. Most dancers, however, realize that a good warm-up is important for reducing the stress of rapid or sudden movements of the joints and for general injury prevention. Not to mention prolonging careers.

Whether or not they like it, as dancers get older their warm-ups usually get longer and longer. The fifteen- to twenty-minute warm-up becomes thirty or forty-five or sixty minutes long. Perhaps younger dancers should also take the time and care to warm up, heeding the words spoken to me once by Erick Hawkins: "Of all the early people in Martha [Graham]'s company, only Merce [Cunningham] and I warmed up, and I warmed up more than Merce and I am dancing more."

The warm-up before a class, rehearsal, or performance is more than a ritual, although for many dancers that may be its primary purpose.[33] In a good warm-up, the dancer increases the core temperature of the body, the heart rate and thus blood flow to the muscles, muscle elasticity, the breathing rate as the diaphragm muscle warms up, and fluid movement into the joints. In addition, the warm-up should increase the sensitivity of the nerve receptors.

What does all this mean in terms of how one spends that fifteen minutes before class or rehearsal? I should first mention that the dancer's warm-up is highly personal. Admittedly, there are dancers who hurl themselves on stage, having just arrived at the theatre, or who walk into company class during pliés, but many dancers would agree that the body and soul have to be prepared in some way for performance—there are, then, some common objectives and characteristics of dance warm-ups.[34] If one wants to dance, one has to be ready to move. The muscles have to be ready. The nervous system has to be ready. The dancer has to be focused on the activity at hand. The movement possibilities for warm-ups are enormous, and dancers have to discover them for themselves (see Inset, next page).

Nonimpact aerobics (NIA) can be used as a dance warm-up—a complete aerobic workout—for modern dance choreography or for stress relief. The dance form is beginning to have substantial impact on the dance world, mainly as a method of conditioning.[35]

Whatever method is used, the warm-up can last anywhere from five minutes to two hours, although twenty to forty minutes seems reasonable for most dancers. The problem is *staying* warm. Teachers give corrections during class. Dancers are rehearsed in groups. Performers have to wait their turn to dance on stage. Frankly, the younger ballerinas can probably get away with sewing satin ribbon onto pointe shoes while they're waiting backstage, at least in the short-run. Eventually, dancing "cold" will catch up with them. Older dancers (here I mean forty-something and above) will probably have to keep moving to keep the core temperature up 1 to 2 degrees.

WHAT SHOULD I BE DOING IN A WARM-UP?: A PRIMER

1. *What: Increase the core temperature, heart rate, blood flow, muscle resiliency, breathing rate.*

   How: Walking, prancing, gentle jogging (springing rather than running), or knee bends—anything that involves a change in level of the body. Even moving the arms, large-arm movements with no flinging, will increase the heart rate. Nonimpact aerobics (NIA) would be especially valuable here. Although the general maxim "Do not stretch to warm up, warm up to stretch" should be followed, once warmed up, there may be some problem areas (e.g., the calf muscles) that are especially tight and need to be stretched before attempting vigorous movement.

2. *What: Lubricate the joints, increase movement of fluid into the joints, although not to the point of overuse.*

   How: Flex and point the toes, ankle circles. Movement of the torso in all directions. Shoulder rolls and drops, arm circles, gentle neck circles (side-to-side). Then, there are the old standards for some dancers: circling the legs in the hip socket, twisting on the floor side-to-side. This is not really helping the muscles much. Chances are these joints will be worked anyway by satisfying "1." above.

3. *What: Focus attention. Try not to fixate on the tight costume, the slippery floor, the clumsy partner, the fight with the sylph or shade next door.*

   How: Think, pray, laugh, sing, meditate. The literature is rich with works on specific methods to enable performers to focus on rehearsal and performance.[a]

4. *What: Neuromuscular patterning, practicing coordination movements and patterns that produce balance, timing, and muscular control necessary for performance.*

   How: Some repetition with attention to dynamic alignment.[b] A ballet barre reinforces needed neuromuscular patterning, especially for complex allegro work. Almost all the ballet and many of the younger modern dancers to whom I speak usually do some barre as part of their warm-up to establish the patterning of movement in the muscles, if nothing else.

[a]See Daniel L. Kohut, *Musical Performance: Learning Theory and Pedagogy* (Englewood Cliffs, N.J.: Prentice-Hall, 1985); Eric W. Krenz, *Gaining Control: Turning Stress into an Asset with Modified Autogenic Training* (Salt Lake City, Utah: I.I.P. Associates, 1983). See also the February 1990 issue of *Journal of Physical Education, Recreation and Dance*, which features six articles on dance and imagery, including creative visualization and enhancing alignment through imagery. This information is useful not only for warming up, but also for training and rehearsal.
[b]See J. Gantz, "Evaluation of faulty dance technique patterns: A working model," *Kinesiology and Medicine for Dance* 12/1 (1989): 1–11.

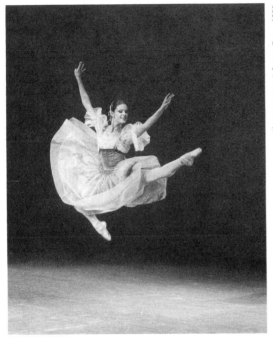

Photo courtesy © Steven Caras, 1990

Merrill Ashley

Merrill Ashley is in many ways a model Balanchine dancer. Tall and leggy with articulate and strong feet, she is well known for her allegro work—her speed, technical skill, attack, and clarity. Unlike Patricia McBride (see profile on page 25), she has worked her way up through the ranks of NYCB, having been awarded principal status nine years after joining the corps. Having reached that point, she has no short-term plans to retire. Says Ashley, "I intend to continue dancing for a long time, if my body permits me to." Hopefully, she will be thrilling audiences with her dazzling footwork well into her forties and beyond.

In *Dancing for Balanchine*,[36] she writes about the hard-won trajectory her career has taken at NYCB. She was "out" much of the time with injuries in her first and second years with the company. She talks about the creative genius of Balanchine, the ballets that were created for her, and the inevitable injuries associated with those ballets—the chronic tendinitis while rehearsing for *Divertimento No. 15*, the ankle sprain when videotaping *Ballo della Regina*, and the sharp hip pain after the premiere of *Ballade* (Dr. Eivind Thomasen eventually performed surgery to relieve pressure on a nerve).

Some of her injuries can be traced to anatomical limitations. For example, the big toe of her left foot is much longer than the other phalanges, and the weight is not evenly distributed on all of them. This causes inflammation of the metatarsal joints of the big toe. But the important point she makes in her book is that the injuries must be taken as an opportunity to retrain the body. Certainly the pressures of professional dance are intense, but "recovery time" can be used to take stock of where one is and what one wants to do with a career.

> When I am injured and have more free time than I am accustomed to, I find myself trying to form a clearer picture in my mind of what I want the overall effect of my dancing to be. . . . The improvement after long layoffs is due not only to the benefits I have derived from "starting from scratch" or from observing others. During a period of recovery, all dancers are forced to be sensitive to the condition and the needs of their bodies in order to make important decisions about which therapies to try or which advice to listen to. . . . After an injury, a dancer learns, at least for a short time, to heed his body if only because pain speaks a language almost anyone can understand. This heightened awareness should not disappear once the dancer returns to form; rather it should help him continue to learn about the ways his body moves and reacts.[37]

This is also a time to evaluate workload and repertory. Sometimes Ashley danced *Ballo della Regina* and *Piano Concerto*, or *Square Dance* and *Theme and Variations* on the same program. In fact, for three-and-one-half years, until 1980, she danced as many as twelve ballets each week. She finally realized, reluctantly, that the key to avoiding frequent injuries was to cut back on the number of performances and/or ballets she did each week.

This point, although seemingly obvious, is advice that should be given to young dancers. At the very least, dancers should be clear about which ballets are the most taxing for their bodies. For example, in *Sleeping Beauty* and *Swan Lake* the body is square and correct alignment is maintained. This is not always the case in abstract works and, for Ashley, injuries are more likely to occur in the nonclassical ballets. She is now able to have a say in whether or not a particular ballet will be included in or taken out of her repertory.

Ashley also feels that she does not automatically have to do every step given in class. She carefully monitors her physical condition and bases her classroom efforts on what she feels capable of on a given day. There are certain types of steps she would venture to try only if she was feeling at her "very best." Ashley says, "All of this makes obvious good sense. But ambition and the dictates of tradition make dancers act otherwise."

. . . .

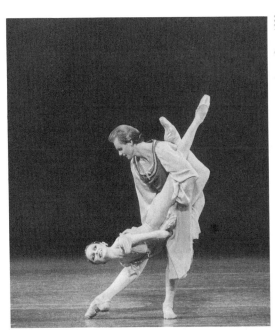

Photo courtesy © Steven Caras, 1990

Adam Lüders

Adam Lüders has been a professional dancer for more than twenty years. Most of his career has been spent as a principal dancer with NYCB, which he was invited to join by the late George Balanchine. Prior to entering NYCB, Lüders—who was born in Denmark and trained at the Royal Danish Ballet School—danced with the Royal Danish Ballet from 1968 to 1973 and the London Festival Ballet (now called English National Ballet) from 1973 to 1975.

For Lüders, "being a dancer means that you use your brain more than you use your legs." He believes that mindless repetition of movement is not an end in itself, but that "it's a means to achieving the physical facility that will eventually permit the dancer to transcend mere physical movement and enter the realm of artistic expression." Technique, Lüders believes, is valuable because it "sets a dancer free to go beyond craftsmanship to artistic expression":

> Dancers need to question what they are doing, not for the sake of being contrary, but because they need to *understand* what they're doing. Movement without meaning, no matter how well executed, is simply athletic display. Most importantly, dancers must take care of themselves. This means taking personal initiative and responsibility, both on stage and off, being guided by choreographers, teachers and other dancers, but also integrating their influences into one's own sensibility.

Lüders often gives himself class, and believes in treating his own injuries whenever possible. He doesn't rush to masseurs or chiropractors—you have to be smart to "handle things for yourself."

Lüders is less worried about injuries—though he has had his fair share—than about the psychological stress of performing. He is the first to admit that the life of the professional dancer is often difficult: "I suffer with my dancing, I'm nervous. I want every performance to be better than the one before; performance is everything to me. When one performance is not as good as another, I am crushed."

And what of his injuries? His arches are exceptionally high and as a result he has always had foot and ankle problems. He has undergone surgery several times, shortening one of the arches in his foot and removing scar tissue that caused chronic inflammation. In both cases, Dr. Eivind Thomasen performed the surgery (see Bibliography for Dr. Thomasen's works). But the chronic inflammation is still there, and recently Lüders has developed some lower-back strain. His body is very tired. But he continues to be everybody's danseur noble.

> Some day it will all be memories, so I am willing to sacrifice that good bottle of wine, my hours of free time, a carelessness about the body that people in less physical professions take for granted. The situation with Ib Anderson and myself is a difficult one—for a long time there were no other principal men in the company and we were dancing all the time. Under those conditions you get overworked, fatigued, injured; you want to scream, but you still go on.

· · · · · · · · · · · · · · · · ·

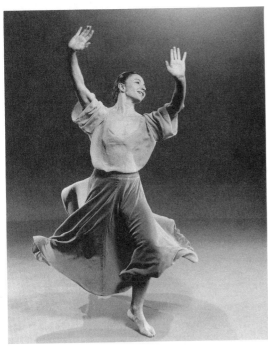

Photo © Johan Elbers, 1990

Risa Steinberg

When Risa Steinberg was a little girl, her family called her Sarah Bernhardt. At age forty, she still engaged audiences with her dramatic stage presence and stunning musicality. Steinberg was born to dance and perform. That doesn't mean that she has had an easy stage life.

A graduate of the High School of Performing Arts and the Juilliard School in New York, Steinberg had trained primarily as a Graham dancer. This was during the time that modern dancers slavishly adhered to (or were supposed to adhere to) a particular "technique" or style of dance: Graham dancers took Graham technique class; Cunningham dancers took Cunningham technique class.

Only five months after graduation from Juilliard, Steinberg had major surgery to repair a herniated disc in her lower back. After the surgery, she stopped by the Juilliard School to say hello to dance department director Martha Hill, and received an unexpected invitation: José Limón was in the office and asked her to come to a rehearsal. She was sure he wasn't serious—after all, she was a *Graham* dancer—but she decided to go anyway.

Steinberg joined Limón's company and danced with him for eleven years. She also performed with the companies of Anna

Sokolow, Daniel Lewis, and Bill Cratty. Now internationally known as a reconstructor of Limón works, she also teaches his technique and is on the dance faculty of the Juilliard School and the Limón school. She performs regularly with Annabelle Gamson, Dance Solos, Inc.

It's an exhausting life. She says, "You have to enjoy it because it's just too hard, the competition is intense and the work is sporadic." However, she easily finds work, touring at least six months each year. Her work is her life: "I am much better if I am working constantly—thinking, moving—I get scared that I won't dance enough, that I'll feel unchallenged and will lose it all."

On top of the chronic overuse injuries that come from working so much, she has also suffered acute injury—tearing the cartilage and tendon in her right shoulder when dancing in Israel. Her most serious injury results from a congenital lower back problem. "I figured I was good for five years with my surgery." Her vertebral discs are fusing, but at least she knows the signs of the pain: "The pain is a warning, a warning to work differently. At least I am not a victim of the pain in that I know how to control it from becoming worse."

For Steinberg, pain and injury tell her that she needs to listen and work differently—usually by seeking different "healers" and therapies that enable her to keep working as a professional dancer: "I am a sponge, if something feels right, I'll absorb it—Pilates, Nautilus, floating in a deprivation tank, massage, acupuncture."

Despite the exhausting performing and teaching schedules, and the physical and emotional challenge of reconstructing Limón's work, she does take the time to heal her mind and body. She listens to her body and to "what it wants and needs to do."

She doesn't have to touch her head to her knees or show a "perfect" arabesque in the repertory she performs. This doesn't make her worse as a dancer. She knows she doesn't have to be on stage with fifteen other people with perfectly turned-out and angled arabesques. But she never did—that's not the life she chose for herself.

> As long as you have something to say, you'll keep performing, even if that means doing things differently. You just adjust. For example, the things inside José [Limón] that he wanted to say no longer demanded him to jump grand jumps, so the roles that he created for himself like the Moor in *The Moor's Pavane* physically didn't demand from him in the same way. I believe that what you say as a dancer when you're thirty-eight and

forty-eight and fifty-eight is very different from what you say when you're eighteen or twenty or twenty-five. What I can dance now I could have never danced when I was eighteen. I would not have known how, nor would I have wanted to.

Three

Technique and Training

A dictionary definition of dance "technique" might be the way in which a dancer uses basic physical movements in performance or the ability to use fundamental physical movements effectively. In casual usage, "technique" has come to refer to a style of dance movement or movement vocabulary. The names associated with techniques are often those of a particular teacher or choreographer—Cecchetti, Bournonville, Hawkins, Cunningham, or Luigi.

The origins of the different techniques vary with the dance idiom. Discussion of them is beyond the scope of this book, but conceptually they represent branches of a tree, rather than steps of a ladder, with no one technique necessarily more progressive or "advanced" than another.

In terms of minimizing injuries and maximizing career longevity, good technique is critical. Some would argue it is of primary importance in keeping the dancer injury-free.

According to Stuart Wright, "The simple fact is that virtually all dance injuries result from faulty technique. . . . Technical correction is the best means to prevention and treatment."[1] Perhaps overstating the case, Wright's point is nevertheless well taken. Dancers rarely have perfect alignment, thus harmful compensations in the weight-bearing joints are likely to occur. Some of the structural limitations resulting in faulty technique and harmful compensations are discussed in greater detail below.

Performing Movement Correctly

Dancers must acquire technique to perform movement in a correct and aesthetically pleasing way, but first they must understand what is needed to perform the movement. This should involve far more than brute repetition of exercises in "technique" classes—taking class on a regular basis, at least for the beginning dancer, is only a first step.[2]

For example, those who have taken Graham classes know that central to the technique is the stylized abdominal contraction, with the head falling backward in hyperextension and the arms reaching forward, wrists hyperextended and fingers flexed. Casual observation in class reveals that the lower torso takes on a concave form when performing the contraction. Verbal cues by the teacher indicate to the student that the abdominal musculature first "releases" and then "contracts."

To execute the movement correctly and safely, however, there should be no anatomical variations (especially in the lower spine) that would interfere with the range of motion required to perform the movement. Furthermore, certain breathing patterns should be used to successfully engage the muscles needed to support the spine.[3]

In short, dancers must have some intuitive, if not formal, knowledge of movement mechanics. (To argue for a more scientific understanding of dance movement is not to deny the equally important spiritual understanding that dancers should bring to their art.) This doesn't mean that dancers have to know the name, origin, and insertion of every muscle in the body. However, it can only improve performance and health to know, for example, that a tight psoas muscle pulls the lower spine into hyperextension, ultimately interfering with the correct alignment of the pelvis and lower body joints because the muscle is attached to all of the lumbar vertebrae and the lowest thoracic.

The dancers whose stories are profiled at the end of this chapter have, for the most part, been self-taught in principles of human structure and movement. For them, and for many in dance, it is technique in the broad sense—information gathering, problem solving—that interests them, rather than technique that narrowly refers to a particular style of dance.

If technique is discovery and mastery of basic principles of movement, then evaluation of technique should involve a physical (i.e., using the principles of physics), or biomechanical, analysis and a structural/functional evaluation. Examples of each are given below. Admittedly, there is far more to understanding dance than performing a physical analysis of component movements. Nevertheless, it serves as an important first step. According to the physicist and dancer Kenneth Laws:

> Certainly ballet cannot be "reduced to a science." But the world of dance is large and complex, with many windows through which one can both perceive and illuminate. . . . [The] view through the window of physical analysis will enhance, not detract from, an appreciation of this art form [and] contribute to the advancement of the art and skill of dance."[4]

Biomechanical Analysis

Human movement has been studied as a science for over two millennia, beginning with the work of Aristotle. Today, "biomechanics" generally concerns itself with principles and laws of mechanics applied to the function of living organisms, usually using quantitative data. It is distinguished from the term "kinesiology" in that kinesiology includes both qualitative and quantitative analysis of human movement and requires thorough knowledge of the neuromuscular system.[5]

One of the first full-length works in the field of dance kinesiology was published in 1984 by Schirmer Books. The strength of *The Physics of Dance* lies in the clear and nontechnical terms that author Kenneth Laws uses to describe how physical laws affect dance movement. With his classic work as a departure, the following discussion is meant to introduce the reader to the language and the power of the analysis.

Plié

The plié is a movement central to most dance forms. It is one of the first movements taught in technique class; anatomically, it is one of the most difficult to execute. To perform it correctly, students must pay attention to the proper alignment of the hip, knee, and ankle joints. As students begin the plié, the legs must be aligned so that a straight line could be drawn from the hip socket through the knee and ankle joints and to the second toe (Fig. 14). This means that the knee should not protrude in front of the toes as judged when looking directly at the toes.

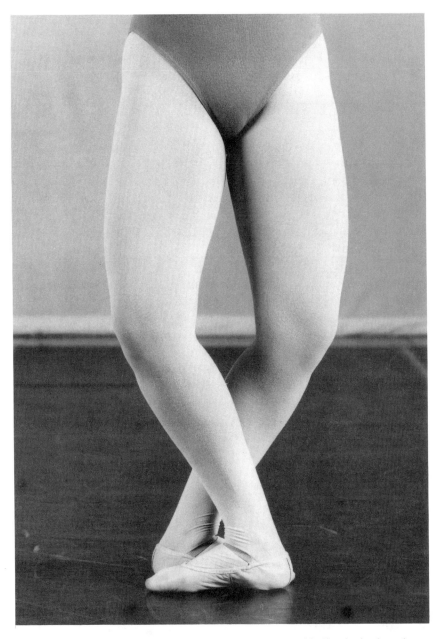

Figure 14. Demi-plié in fifth position. Ideally, in classical ballet the heels and toes should be touching. *(Photo by Anthony Hall)*

It takes time to develop a serviceable plié. Dance students are too concerned with *results*, but acquiring good technique is a lifetime process.[6]

PIROUETTE

Understanding the mechanism by which a torque (see Medical and Technical Glossary) is exerted against the floor can enhance dancers' ability to control any turn performed on one leg. A torque is exerted by the body on the floor to initiate a pirouette. The reaction torque of the floor on the body actually causes the body to start turning.[7]

To execute a successful pirouette, dancers have to stretch vertically, pushing into the floor with the supporting foot, while reaching for the ceiling through the top of the head. The dancers are actually exerting a torque against the floor by pushing in a horizontal direction with one foot and the opposite direction with the other, with some distance between the feet.

The more vertical the body, the easier the turn because for a given magnitude of angular momentum (or quantity of angular motion), if the moment of inertia is small (i.e., the mass of the body is close to the rotation axis), the rate of turn will be relatively large and hence less effort will be required to produce it. An off-center mass will wobble around the rotation axis, creating an unstable situation (Fig. 15). If the body is not well aligned (i.e., part of the body is "off axis," as when the arms are held too far forward), centrifugal force will tend to increase the body's distance from the axis of rotation. This means that the supporting leg also will move around the rotation axis, turning with a wobble. As a result, the turn is much less smooth and more difficult.

JUMPS

Many aspects of jumps can be submitted to physical analysis. Much of Laws' *The Physics of Dance* is devoted to their discussion. For example, he describes at some length the "floating illusion" during a traveling jump such as a grand jeté. Aesthetically, this "illusion" is very desirable because the dancer appears to be floating horizontally near the peak of the jump before beginning the descent. The dancer appears almost to defy gravity, in part because the vertical motion of the body is quick at the beginning and end of the jump, but slow near the peak. (According to equations of projectile motion, one-half of the total time the body is in the air is spent within one-quarter of the

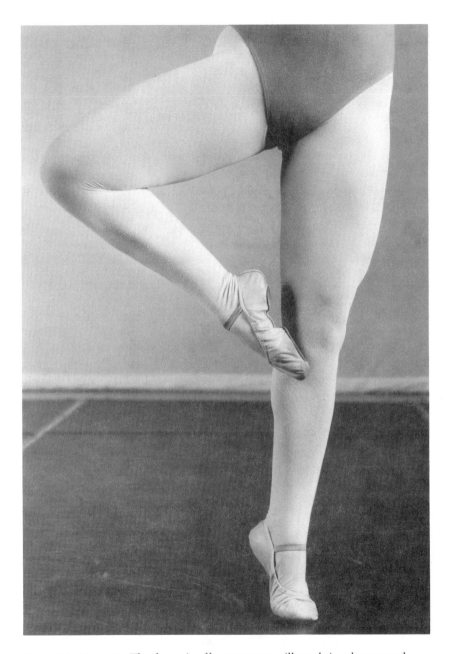

Figure 15. Pirouette. The dancer's off-center mass will result in a less smooth, wobbly turn. *(Photo by Anthony Hall)*

height to the peak of the jump.) Control of body configuration while in flight can enhance this illusion even more.

Once the magnitude and direction of the initial velocity upon leaving the floor are determined, the shape of the parabolic trajectory followed by the center of gravity can be predicted. Although the dancer cannot change this trajectory in flight, the relative position of the body's center of gravity (indicated by the letter "O" in Figure 16a) can be changed by controlling the body configuration.

For example, lifting the arms and legs near the peak of the jump (Fig. 16b) causes the position of the center of gravity in the body to rise. If that rise and subsequent descent of the center of gravity relative to the body coincides with the rise and fall of the center of gravity in its trajectory in space, then the head and torso can actually move horizontally for a short time, creating the illusion of floating.[8] Rhonda Ryman, in a kinematic analysis of grand allegro jumps (see Bibliography), makes the point that the height of the jump is not completely dependent on the depth of the preceding plié, since a very deep knee bend can cause a mechanical disadvantage at the knee joint.

LIFTS

Lifting involves a partnership between two or more dancers—a partnership that involves trust and responsibility. For purposes of brevity and clarity of discussion, I will assume the person lifting is male and the person being lifted is female. The woman trusts that her partner will control her descent to the floor. Likewise, the man trusts that his partner will carefully time her jump so that part of the upward impetus comes from the jump, not solely from his strength. The woman must maintain a vertical body configuration to assist as much as possible in the lift.

Each partner has a responsibility to develop the coordination that will allow both of them to use their strength effectively in a supported pose. If each partner is not sensitive to the timing, balance, and strength needed to successfully execute a lift, injuries may result. As stated by Kenneth Laws:

> Controlling a non-rigid weight equal to perhaps three-fourths of [the male's] own weight can be tricky and demanding. For high lifts, his back takes substantial compressive stress, particularly in the lumbar region when its curvature is exaggerated. Since the woman's weight is often borne by the man's hands, the position of the hands is important in avoiding unnecessary stress. If his arms are not vertical [especially in a sustained lift], there is

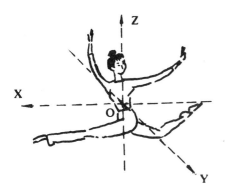

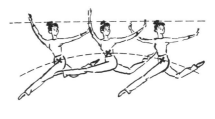

a. "O" marks the location of the center of gravity.

b. The relative position of the center of gravity is changed by lifting the arms and legs toward the peak of the trajectory, creating the illusion that the head and torso have moved horizontally.

Figure 16. Physical analysis of the "floating illusion" common to many classical ballet forms. (*Adapted from Kenneth Laws,* The Physics of Dance. *New York: Schirmer Books, 1984, p. 35*)

substantial torque in the shoulders with possible muscle or tendon injury.[9]

The *vertical lift* is decidedly easier to accomplish if the woman who is being lifted does not have to reach a stable equilibrium position during the lift. When the choreography does require that the lift be "held," the combined center of gravity of the two people must be directly over the area of support. For example, in Figure 17*a*, the woman is slightly "bending at the waist" at the peak of the jump. Her center of gravity is thus displaced forward, producing a torque that tends to rotate her upper body forward, a more difficult position for her partner to sustain. The lifter then compensates by hyperextending his lower spine near the peak of the lift.

Figure 17*b* shows the correct body configuration for a vertical lift. Close to the peak of the lift, the lifter should fully extend the arms and legs, thus increasing the force they can exert.[10] Note that the woman's body is "straight," her center of gravity is in the same vertical line as her partner's, and thus the force he exerts is almost entirely vertical.

Also important to the success of the lift is the proper positioning of the hands and the distance between the two partners. In the straight vertical lift, support is provided with the heel of the hand directly underneath the rib cage, so that the base of the rib cage receives much of the vertical supporting force (Fig. 18*b*), not with the fingers and

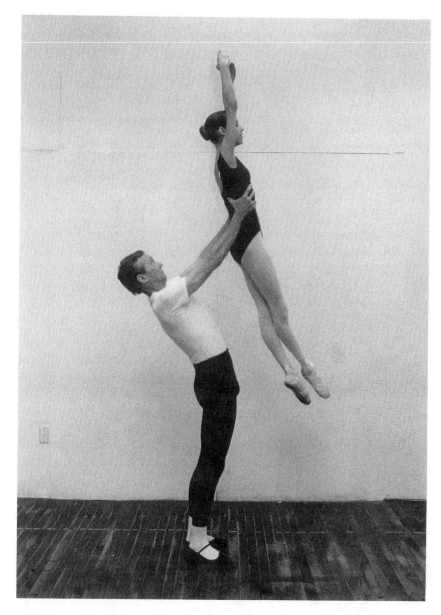

a. Incorrect: lifter shows extreme lumbar hyperextension as the woman bends forward from the waist.

Figure 17. Vertical lift. Kenneth Laws and Cathleen Fischbach of the Central Pennsylvania Youth Ballet. *(Photos by A. Pierce Bounds)*

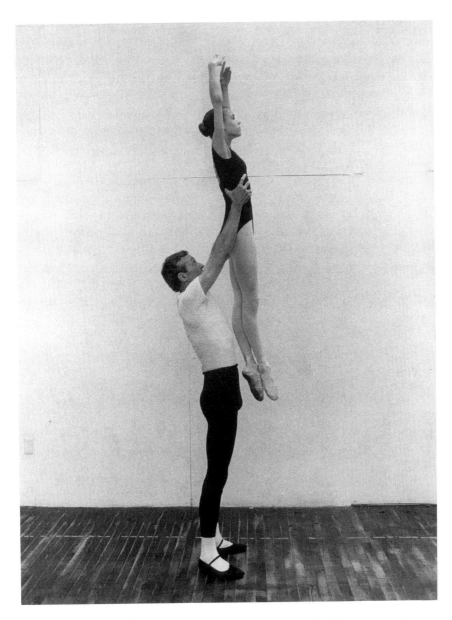

b. Correct: showing only slight lumbar hyperextension in the lifter's spine; the woman's body configuration is almost completely vertical.

thumbs squeezing between the ribs and the hip bones (Fig. 18a). Inexperience usually causes the full weight of the woman to be supported by her partner's thumbs, thus leading to sprains and strains. Note also in Figure 18a that the elbows are more extended than in Figure 18b, thus rendering the torque in the shoulders very large (approximately a force of 1,100 pounds in the muscle-tendon system of each shoulder) and possibly resulting in injury.

In general, the distance between the two partners should be less rather than more. If the lift is initiated at too great a distance, there is a large torque at the hip joint exerted by the muscles attached to the lower back. The greater distance between the partners in Figure 18a forces the man to use his upper back and shoulder muscles to support the lift, thus adding stress to the spine. Ideally, the large muscle groups of the hips and legs (the gluteus maximus and quadriceps, respectively) should be used, together with the shoulder flexors and elbow extensors.

In the *arabesque lift*, as with lifts in general, the tendency for the woman to rotate or rock backward in a clockwise direction must be

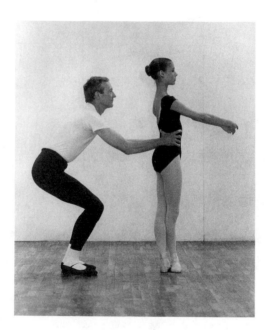

a. Vertical lift (incorrect)

Figure 18. Positioning of the hands in lifts. Kenneth Laws and Cathleen Fischbach of the Central Pennsylvania Youth Ballet. *(Photos by A. Pierce Bounds)*

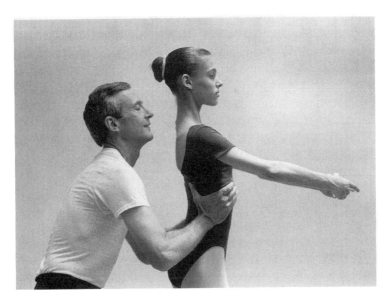

b. Vertical lift (correct)

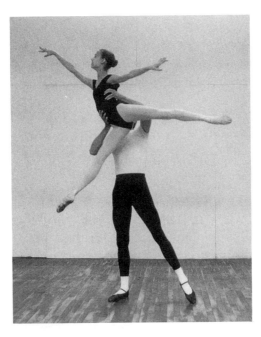

c. Arabesque lift (correct)

counteracted by a torque. The torque is exerted by pushing her upper back forward with the downstage (left) hand and pushing her hips backward with the upstage (right) hand (Fig. 18c). The left hand must be held high on the body with the left thumb around the shoulder blade; the weight, however, is mostly borne by the right hand. The elbow of the right arm must be held close to the body in order to engage more of the abdominal muscles. The left elbow is then lifted to engage the front-shoulder (anterior deltoid) muscles to push the upper body forward. In addition, the erector spinae muscles should be used to support the trunk during lifts.

Structural and Functional Analysis

There are a number of anatomical variations that limit the dancer's ability to perform a movement correctly. The following are a few examples of structural constraints that some dancers may face in the foot, ankle, and hip.[11] Dancers usually have to find outside help—an orthopedist, podiatrist, kinesiologist, physical therapist, coach, or paraprofessional with training in anatomy and kinesiology—to assist in evaluation of the structural variation. Functional constraints (weak, tight muscles and muscle imbalances) are also considered in the discussion below.

FOOT AND ANKLE

There are a number of common anatomical variations in the foot and ankle that predispose a dancer to injury. One example of this is the presence of a small bone, the os trigonum, at the back of the talus. When fused with the talus, it appears as a protrusion or process. If separated from the talus, it appears as a separate bone.

Whether fused or not, its presence easily restricts plantar flexion. As dancers assume a full-pointe position, there may be soft tissue irritation and inflammation. Some dancers with this condition may be asymptomatic, but may compensate by sickling the foot to appear higher on pointe. Unfortunately, this overstretches the outside foot and ankle tendons as the foot rolls out (Fig. 19).

Dancers who have a high instep and somewhat rigid foot structure may also have a tendency to roll their feet to the outside, overstretching the outside tendons. Furthermore, the more rigid the foot structure and the more tightly the joint is held together, the less shock absorption is possible in the muscles of the joint.

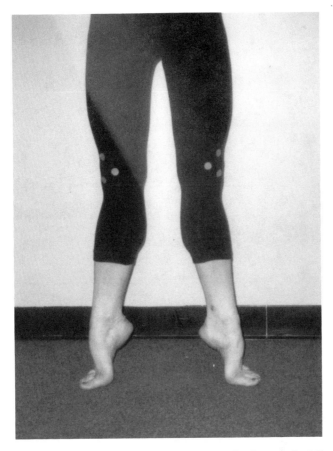

Figure 19. Sickling the right foot in relevé. The desired "look" is to increase the height of the relevé; the effect is to stretch the outside foot and ankle tendons as the foot rolls out. *(Photo by Marika Molnar, P.T.)*

For the foot with an unusually high longitudinal arch, the toes appear clawed and heavy calluses may form on the top of the toes. Abnormal stresses are placed on the instep, the ball of the foot, and the heel. The dancer may be asymptomatic, but when pain does occur it will result from pressure put on the metatarsals. In either of these cases dancers may find that motion is not restricted and that there is little pain upon movement. However, they should be aware of any harmful compensations that may be occurring in other parts of the body.

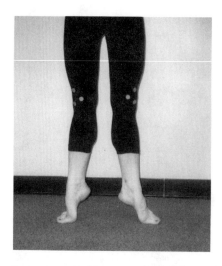

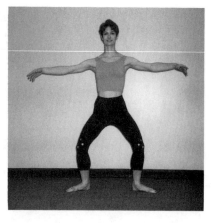

Figure 20a. Rolling in on the left foot, which overstretches the inside foot and ankle tendons. *(Photos by Marika Molnar, P.T.)*

Figure 20b. In this second position demi-plié, dancer Barbara Gagas is rolling in with both feet, stressing the inside foot and ankle tendons. In addition, her pelvis has an anterior tilt as she forces rotation at the knee joint.

HIP: EXTERNAL ROTATION

External rotation at the hip is desirable in most Western dance forms, but classical ballet in particular emphasizes "perfect turnout." However, one would need a slightly imperfect anatomy to achieve this perfect turnout of 90 degrees at each hip. Usually no more than 60 to 70 degrees can be derived from external rotation at the hip, the remainder achieved at the expense of forcing outward rotation of the knee and the foot and ankle.

A number of structural factors influence the amount of external hip rotation that is possible, including the angle of femoral anteversion (easily seen in dancers whose kneecaps seem to face inward when feet are in parallel position), orientation of the acetabulum relative to the femur, elasticity of the anterior hip capsule, and flexibility of the muscle-tendon units that cross the hip joint.

Dancers frequently compensate for inadequate hip turnout by winging or rolling in on the foot (Fig. 20a). Instead of turning out at the hip joint, they overutilize the outside leg and ankle muscles to achieve the turnout. The same compensation occurs in second position demi-plié (Fig. 20b): the foot is forced to stretch along the inside border, which strains the structures of the medial foot and knee.

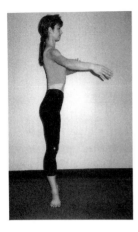

Figure 21a. Incorrect
alignment showing anterior
pelvic tilt and feet excessively
"turned out." *(Photos by
Marika Molnar, P.T.)*

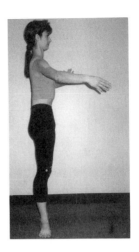

Figure 21b. Incorrect
alignment showing posterior
pelvic tilt and feet excessively
"turned out."

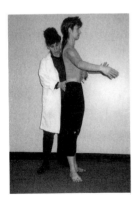

Figure 21c. Marika Molnar
corrects the dancer's alignment
by adjusting the position
of the pelvis.

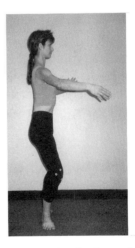

Figure 21d. The dancer is
maintaining a neutral position
of the pelvis while performing
a demi-plié.

Rolling in on the foot is usually accompanied by adjustments in the pelvis. The pelvis may be tilted so that the natural curve of the lumbar spine is exaggerated in an anterior pelvic tilt (Fig. 21*a*) or flattened in a posterior pelvic tilt, or "tucking" (Fig. 21*b*). In Figure 21*c*, physical therapist Marika Molnar corrects the alignment by adjusting the position of the pelvis and reducing the motion at the foot. In Figure 21*d*, the dancer maintains a neutral position of the pelvis while performing a demi-plié. The tendency, however, is still to "anchor" the foot and rotate from the knees in a plié position.

A *test for hip external rotation* conducted by Marika Molnar is shown in Figure 22*a*. Full turnout is achieved by rotation from the knee in plié—this is not advised because of the resulting stress (torque) that occurs as the legs are straightened. By observing the position of the markers on the kneecap, one can see how turnout increases slightly when the dancer flexes her hips (Fig. 22*b*).

The exercise shown in Figure 22*c* also tests for turnout. If the external rotators are weak and/or the latissimus dorsi muscle is tight, the lumbar spine will be drawn into hyperextension, as shown.

Karen Clippinger-Robertson has carefully outlined a series of tests for flexibility.[12] Since proper measurement is essential for accurate results, she uses a goniometer—a device that measures the angle between different body segments. The test requires that subjects lie on their back with both hips extended and knees straight, externally rotating one leg from the hip joint. The end point of the stable arm of the goniometer must be in contact with the midpoint of the kneecap. The number of degrees that the femur can be outwardly rotated from this starting position is measured in positive degrees. Some experts recommend a minimum of 60 degrees for classical ballet dancers.

Hip: extension

In Figure 23*a*, the dancer extends her leg to the back using primarily lumbar spine extension, rather than available hip extension. She tilts the top of the pelvis forward so that the iliofemoral ligament and the iliopsoas slacken and the lower back hyperextends. This compensation places stress on the lower spine and slackens the structures that actually should be stretched. Figure 23*b* shows acceptable alignment during the tendu derrière, the hip flexors allowing free movement to the back without substituting back extension and the abdominals bracing and supporting the lumbar spine.

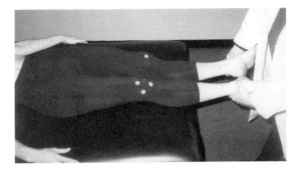

a. The dancer's turnout on the right side is somewhat limited.

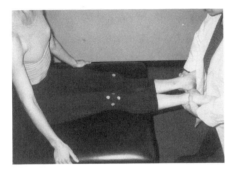

b. Turnout increases slightly on the right leg when the dancer is in hip flexion.

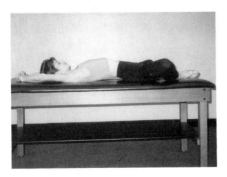

c. The dancer must use the external rotators of the hip to press the thighs downward.

Figure 22. Testing for external hip rotation. *(Photos by Marika Molnar, P.T.)*

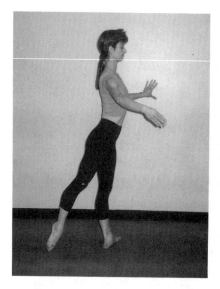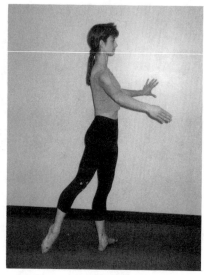

a. Tendu derrière, tilting the pelvis forward.

b. Tendu derrière, neutral pelvis.

Figure 23. Hip extension. *(Photos by Marika Molnar, P.T.)*

In a *test for hip extension,* it may be necessary to isolate the hip extension action (Fig. 24) in order to find the range of motion. In the tests that Karen Clippinger-Robertson has developed, subjects lie on their back at the edge of a table, bringing both knees to the chest and then lowering one leg back toward the table while the knee remains flexed. The position is similar to that shown in Figure 24; the difference is that the hands hold the leg in front of the knee rather than behind it. Zero degrees on the goniometer refers to the position when the leg is lying flat on the table. The number of degrees (at least +30 for dancers) the leg can be brought past the table is then measured. If the hip flexors are so tight that the thigh can't even touch the table, the angle is recorded as negative degrees.

Choosing a Teacher

Learning good dance technique can be a complex process given the presuppositions, biases, or history the student brings to an instructional setting. Key, however, to that setting is the teacher, and in particular, teacher-student relations. The teacher plays many roles in

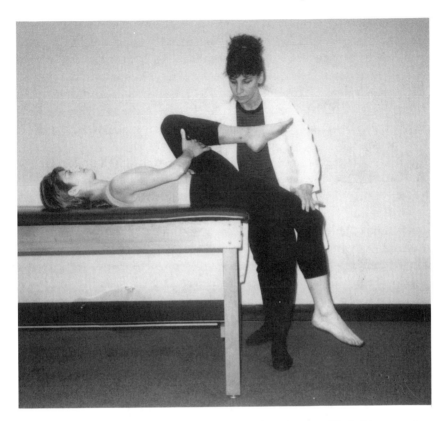

Figure 24. Marika Molnar measures the range of motion possible in hip extension. *(Photo by Marika Molnar, P.T.)*

the dancer's life—mentor, coach, critic, healer, friend—often, too many roles.

Traditionally, correction (and assessment) of technique remained the domain of dance teachers who were not always educated in anatomy and movement mechanics, who could not advise on injury prevention and treatment. But, Judy Gantz notes, "Today, this process is more frequently carried out by dance specialists who have both a dance-science and dance-training background, such as dance kinesiologists, physical therapists, and dance-medicine professionals."[13]

Dancers should be critical and selective consumers. This may be difficult, especially in smaller cities and rural areas, where selecting a good teacher might mean long commutes and considerable expense. It is often worth it. Rather than a teacher who merely shows particular steps, students must find one who can explain *why* a particular step needs to be done. They need a teacher who motivates them to challenge their individual abilities—irrespective of age and career goals—and who helps them to develop their creative and expressive talents. This is a tall order. As a Limón technique teacher once said to me, "You move across that floor as if it were your last time. Believe me, as you get older, *no one* cares if you move or not except you."

A good teacher, besides being competent and knowledgeable, should facilitate the guided self-discovery so important to the growth of the student as dancer and artist. In such a safe and nurturing environment, students will learn to develop movement that is aesthetically pleasing as well as anatomically sound, eventually becoming their own teachers.

Younger dancers must be able to recognize and avoid a teacher who is long on criticism, short on clear explanations, and who humiliates students repeatedly. They must look for a teacher who allows meaningful dialogue and mutual exchange.[14]

Perhaps the best way to identify good teaching is to be critical of the exercises that are taught.

- Is each exercise purposeful?
- Is there a reason for performing the movement?
- Is the *teacher* well informed on the movement intent? In ballet, petite batterie is used to prepare the dancer for the much larger beating steps that are performed at higher elevations. This may be an obvious example of why a certain movement is done in class. Perhaps less obvious is why a ballet class usually starts with grand plié.
- Why stretch the hamstrings at the barre by rounding the back and bringing the head to the knee instead of pressing the lower back into the leg (exercises should emphasize spinal extension rather than flexion—we spend much of our lives resting/ slouching/relaxing in spinal flexion with the same muscles repeatedly tightened or stretched)?
- Why does a modern dance class emphasize swings in the early segments of the class, emphasize exercises with hip flexion, and neglect stretches for the hip flexors?

The correct answer to all these questions is not "Because it feels good," "Because we've always done it," or "Because the teacher says so." As Erick Hawkins says, "You have to act on some *principles* of movement." It is the teacher's responsibility to point out to the student exactly what those principles are and how they should be applied. The movement must make real kinesiological/anatomical sense. Otherwise, it may serve no useful purpose other than as a harmless (or not-so-harmless) diversion.

Older Dancers: Studying with the Best or Not at All

The older dancers I have interviewed are quick to argue that finding good teachers is of primary importance in mastering good technique and extending performing careers. Usually, they are their own best teachers: very careful when they take classes with others and considering very carefully what they are asked to do. Wendy Perron commented, "I won't go to a class now if the teacher picks on me . . . even yoga and t'ai chi (where one has to stay in demi-plié)."

Some have turned to the body therapies (see page 41) not only for technical training and retraining, but also for rehabilitation from injury. Fortunately, the body therapies are appearing in more and more curricula, so that younger professional dancers are exposed to them. They learn body therapies in performing arts high schools, in colleges and universities, and at dance festivals (e.g., the American Dance Festival, of which body therapy proponent Martha Myers is dean).

Jan Hyatt (see profile, page 93) has perhaps summed up the feelings of many dancers:

> As a dancer, you simply need to take responsibility for your body. You need to have intelligent training and you need to be connected with your physical instrument. You need to listen to it and not abuse it. It's designed to move—to abuse it when it's your instrument of expression just for special effect is stupid. It is not luck that prevents injuries; rather, it is being sentiently connected to what's going on with your body when you are moving. "I am a body," not "I have a body." You must think this not just in technique class but at all times. You can't be abusive with your body one day and make up for it the next. You must study with someone that has true body awareness.

She should know. In northwestern Pennsylvania, she had no choice: she drove 30,000 miles in one year just to find those good teachers.

Profiles

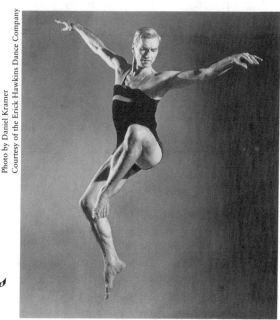

Photo by Daniel Kramer
Courtesy of the Erick Hawkins Dance Company

Erick Hawkins

A native of Colorado, Erick Hawkins came to dance "late," at the age of nineteen. In the sixty years since he first started studying dance, he has been touched by many of dance's leading figures. He was one of Balanchine's first students at the School of American Ballet (SAB). He studied there for four years. He then danced with Martha Graham, becoming her company's first male dancer in 1938 (and later marrying her). It was during his twelve-year tenure with the Graham Company that he began to formulate his technique.

The ease of movement that his technique develops is apparent in his choreography, but more than ease of movement, the dances speak of a great potential for human development. Hawkins's dances celebrate the human spirit—full of hope, beauty, and delight—and eschew the dark and violent side of human nature, which he thinks explains their rather limited appeal. In an interview with Joseph Mazo of the *New York Times*, Hawkins stated:

> I think one reason some people didn't cotton to my work. . . is that they like to see violence of some kind on the stage. Love of violence is immature. In "New Moon," I tried to show what

youth can be, rather than what it too often is. I know that at that stage of my life I was never that unconscious of my actions, but what's happening in the world demonstrates that many people are. The elephants are nearly extinct, our streets are filled with the violent and the homeless—we need a renewal of spiritual insight. [15]

Hawkins is relentless in presenting his aesthetic—steeped in Eastern philosophies, classicism, ritual, and primal experiences—to admittedly small audiences. Part of presenting beauty on the stage is using live music, sculptural design elements, and costumes—all of which give his works their great sensual appeal.

He doesn't seem to have a commercial bone in his body. When asked about any choreographers he might admire, Mark Morris, for example, his reply was, "Yes, I've seen his work, it's good. But it's so hard to keep it pure. We'll see what happens to him."

> I could use chance in my work . . . and other tricks and gimmicks. And I'd have larger audiences. A lot of choreographers out there are just attention-getters. People still give them credit for something that's not there. But that's not how Bartok's works were crafted. They were crafted out of love. Lincoln Kirstein once offered me a commission for a dance for NYCB. How could I do that? I don't approve of ballet, it's so kinesiologically unsound. If I tried to do a popular work, I would lose my audience.

The audiences may be small at concerts, but the classes his company offers are anything but. No doubt it is in his technique or "normative theory of movement" rather than in his choreography that Hawkins will have the largest influence in dance.

In his technique, freedom of movement in the hips is critical to moving efficiently and safely. The abdominal muscles and back extensors must be very strong to support the free-flowing movement in the joints. Such strength also allows for a free-flowing upper torso.

> I've always questioned *why* people move the way they do. To me, the movement must be efficient with no extraneous effort. The greatest beauty in the water is the person who does not splash. How does one achieve this? By honoring principles of kinesiology. You do not force the movement, you allow the movement to happen—always focusing on the thigh socket.

For many years that technique has served him well. However, in

1988, while moving his company from a Manhattan studio to more expansive quarters, Hawkins suffered some inflammation in his ankle. Three months after that move, he suffered a stroke. For the first time since 1935, he was off the stage. Until that time, he had never really been incapacitated. His technique, a steadfast adherence to movement originating in the hip socket, had kept him injury-free.

. . . .

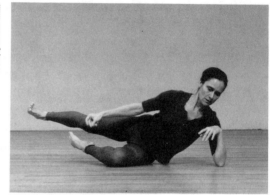

Photo by Jed Downhill

June Finch

June Finch danced with Viola Farber for eight years without missing a single performance. Although at age forty-nine she does not perform with the same intensity as when she was younger, she sees no reason to stop:

> The essence of dancing has nothing to do with biological age. There's such a spirituality that comes with an older age. Look at Merce [Cunningham]! Sure, the kids in his company are leaping and bouncing and I love all that too. I'll leap and turn for as long as I can.

How? With Cecchetti ballet technique—for Finch, it is almost a religion.

Finch has always been considered a Cunningham dancer and teacher, and was teaching for Cunningham when she joined Viola Farber's company. She had been exposed to "all the great styles and techniques" at Sarah Lawrence College, where she received her B.A. and M.A. (studying with Bessie Schönberg), and during summer study at the American Dance Festival in the early 1960s.

It was through Viola Farber, however, that she was first introduced to the soundness of the Cecchetti principles. Cecchetti emphasizes the use of natural alignment as the key to strength and flexibility. From her Cecchetti-oriented teachers she learned to "work *with*, not against, the human body as it is made" (i.e., no gripping, no strain), and began to include these principles in all her teaching. Together with Cunningham technique (or any dance pedagogy), this has proved to be a winning combination for Finch and for her students.

. . . .

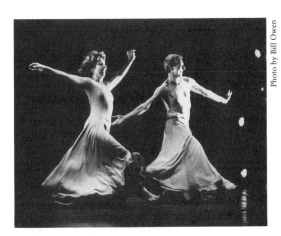

Photo by Bill Owen

Jan Hyatt

For Jan Hyatt, training is everything—it nurtures the dancer's body and soul. But in western Pennsylvania, that training has not been easy to come by. As coordinator of the dance program at Allegheny College in Meadville, she is constantly seeking outside funding for dance residencies so that she and her students can be exposed to diverse modes of training.

She has been successful: Bill Evans has housed his Summer Institute at the College, Gregg Lizenbery has performed at the Institute, and Erick Hawkins has brought his company to the campus. She herself has studied with many other ballet and modern masters.

Hyatt is also willing to commute to find the training she needs. She regularly drives to Pittsburgh (200 miles round trip) to take ballet class. And if a B.A., B.S., M.A., and M.F.A. were not enough, Hyatt is a doctoral candidate in the Arts in Education Program at Teachers

College, Columbia University, still teaching at Allegheny, still writing grant proposals.

All of this is consistent with her general philosophy of information-gathering:

> You have to believe in yourself. I'm fifty-three years old and I wouldn't touch the Graham technique. And if I went to a ballet class and whoever was teaching said that I needed to straighten my legs in fifth position and sacrifice everything for the line, I would leave. You just have to take responsibility for your own body. You have to find the training that is best for it.

Hyatt believes that dancers must train in techniques that do not superimpose an arbitrary skeletal alignment on them. It is the initiation of movement and strengthening the deep abdominal muscles that are important. Strength in the lower torso frees up the movement possibilities. Above all, dancers have to take responsibility for their training:

> You should use dance to relieve stress in your life, performing movement that reduces the risk of injury—not the other way around. Modern dance relies on a live intelligence for communication, you do not need the pyrotechnics. To do a type of dance that adds stress and increases your chances of being injured is silly. You must take responsibility for your training and what you will do and not do. How you move is the key to how long you will move.

• • • • • • • • • • • • • • • •

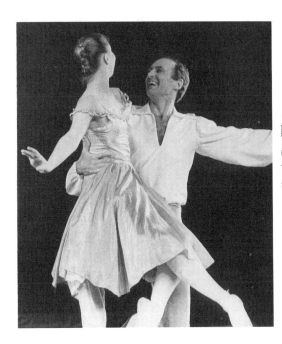

Photo by Tom Wilson
Courtesy of *The Dickinsonian*, Dickinson College

Kenneth Laws

Kenneth Laws, professor of physics at Dickinson College in Carlisle, Pennsylvania, admits that he discovered dance later in life than most people who take it seriously. Dancer, critic, observer, and researcher, Laws analyzes movement so that he can perform and inform dancers everywhere on physical principles that must be acknowledged in a "new pas de deux."

Even after his popular book, *The Physics of Dance*, was published in 1984, Laws has continued to dance, perform, and write on physical principles applied to dance. Quite often, he is asked to partner members of the Central Pennsylvania Youth Ballet (CPYB) in class. In performance, as one of the tallest males in the company, he partners the largest women. He depends heavily on his ability to understand movement through physical analysis to solve problems in partnering and other dance movements.

CPYB is a dance school and a performing company with unusually high standards, spawning a number of talents in the dance world (Lisa de Ribère, Sean Lavery, Tina LeBlanc, and many other dancers in NYCB and ABT). He says, "I have been fortunate to gain acceptance as a rare 'non-youth' in the Youth Ballet, and owe an enormous debt of gratitude to the artistic director, Marcia Dale Weary, and others at the school who have, with remarkable patience, accommodated the unique needs of an older dancer." [16]

Laws, either teaching or taking a pas de deux class, is eager to give corrections to the younger artists. He explains why they are falling off pointe, leaning too far backward into their partners' hands, covering little distance with their grand jeté. His advice is well taken by students all over the country who attend his workshops.

— Four —

The Fit Dancer: Conditioning for Strength, Endurance, and Flexibility

Technique class by itself cannot provide the conditioning necessary for injury-free performance. Dancers need stamina to perform demanding variations, strength to lift other dancers, and flexibility to achieve the aesthetically desired line of many ballet or jazz movements. According to dance kinesiologist Karen Clippinger-Robertson,

> the aesthetically desired line of many dance movements such as a large jump . . . or jazz lay-out requires both great flexibility and strength. . . . intricate pointe [work] require[s] fine neuromuscular coordination. Each of these necessary components [of fitness] should be adequately stressed and developed in dancers' training programs.[1]

Some dancers become so serious about strength training that they are now competitive bodybuilders.[2] Nevertheless, the focus of this chapter is not to encourage dancers to enter posing competitions, but to present principles of conditioning and sample programs so that they can minimize injuries, prolong their performing career, and keep fit once they stop performing.

The programs include conditioning for strength, endurance, and flexibility. They are by no means inclusive of all exercises dancers may want to try; they typify effective conditioning regimens based on principles of dance science and the physical demands of classical and modern choreography. Specific recommendations, considerations, and main points are highlighted in italics throughout the chapter.

Strength

Strength is important for the execution of many dance movements. For example, in Figure 25*a* Nancy Lee's upper-body strength (triceps, deltoid, and pectoral muscles eccentrically contracting) allows her to break the fall carefully. In Figure 25*b*, Glenn Edgerton supports Tina LeBlanc's weight by the strength of his lower-extremity muscles and his trunk extensors.

Figure 26 illustrates some of the compensations dancers make when they do not possess sufficient strength to sustain a grand

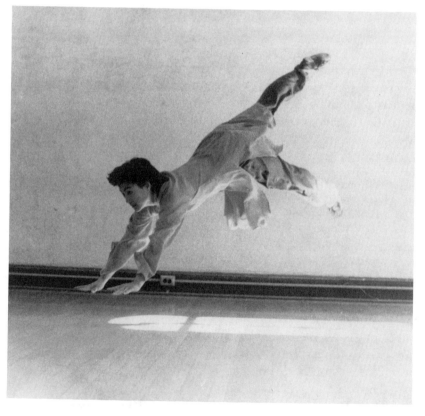

a. Nancy Lee. *(Photo by Peter Affeld)*

Figure 25. Strength on stage.

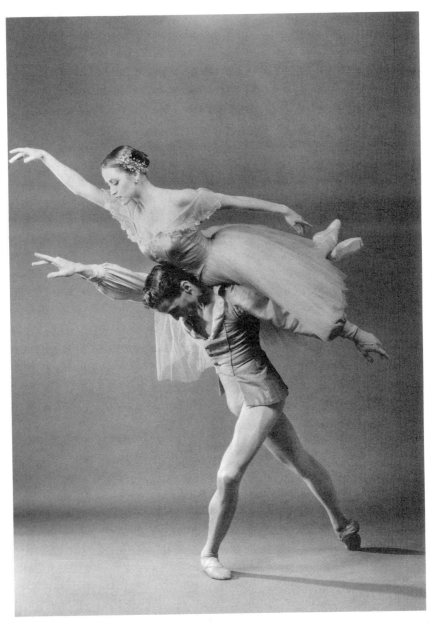

b. Glenn Edgerton partners Tina LeBlanc. *(Photo by Herbert Migdoll. Courtesy of the Joffrey Ballet.)*

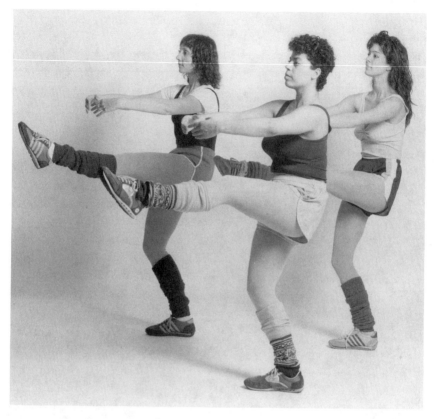

Figure 26. Gigi Berardi, Mirabel Cruz, and Brenna Bond *(left* to *right). (Photo by Bill Owen)*

battement. The dancer in the foreground is flexing the knee of her working leg; the dancer behind her (far right) is leaning backward, "cheating" by flexing the spine to achieve the "look" of high extension (hip flexion). If dancers don't want to make such compensations, their muscles must be sufficiently strong to support the lifted weight. What can they do to achieve this strength?

Former NYCB principal Daniel Duell encourages the lifting of free weights among the dancers he directs in Ballet Chicago. Duell says, "Dancers dance hard for ten or fifteen years and then fall apart physically. Strength training is necessary to prevent this." Lifting free weights is just one way to strength train. There are others: programs that use only body weight for resistance, those that use wall racks or machines, those that use progressively heavier free weights. The type of training programs that are best suited to dancers' needs are addressed throughout this chapter.

Note that all of the programs should be preceded by an adequate warm-up, at least ten minutes on a stationary bicycle, light running in place, or performing movements involving a change in level (e.g., as in nonimpact aerobics). Training sessions should be followed by static or slow stretching to reduce muscle soreness. Some coaches recommend waiting about six hours before stretching; it is a form of recovery that may be counterproductive to the strengthening work.[3]

Strength Training Using Body Weight for Resistance

The work that Kathryn Karipides does is just one example of a regimen that uses body weight as resistance for strengthening. She bases her training methods on movement principles of Scandinavian gymnastics.

Karipides uses this "daily body work" (Figs. 27a–f, 28, and 29) to maintain her level of conditioning. The work helps her to evaluate her dynamic flexibility, coordination, and agility. The body work can also serve as a warm-up or as a centering/focusing exercise for technique class.

Karipides draws on three main sources of movement systems and styles: Emily Andrews of Case Western Reserve University (CWRU), Hanya Holm, and Erick Hawkins. Emily Andrews, director of physical education at CWRU, was a devotee of the gymnastics system developed by Niels Bukh. The system was based on "Danish gymnastics" and is freer in style and range of movement than that allowed by standard Swedish gymnastics.[4]

Karipides gives credit to Hanya Holm for the introduction to a creative kinetic vocabulary and to Erick Hawkins for the training in free-flowing movement. Elements of Hawkins's work can be seen especially in Figure 27f.[5] Karipides believes that "There are universal physical truths that can't be denied. Much of modern technique has added quirks and cosmetics and it's easy to focus on these rather than the basis of the movement—the strength of the pelvic muscles and the alignment of the torso."[6]

The strengthening movement Karipides has developed uses imagery—the ability to imagine fluid shapes and forms that actually affect movement and balance between different muscle groups. She

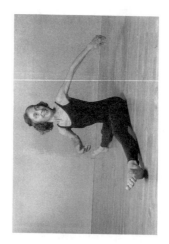

c. In a straddle position, Karipides rotates side-to-side.

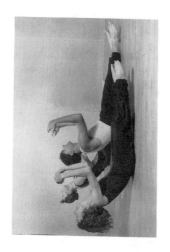

b. Karipides is pictured with students Angela Patrinos (background) and Louis Kavouras (foreground) in a front-and-back "rocking" movement sequence with knees extended (*above*) and flexed (*below*).

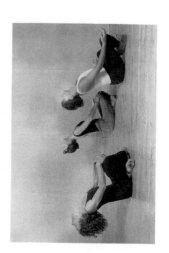

a. Karipides begins her movement sequence rolling side-to-side, front-to-back, after a light warm-up.

Figure 27. Kathryn Karipides' daily strengthening regimen. *(Photos by Mike Sands)*

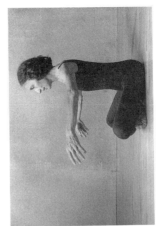

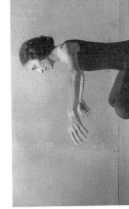

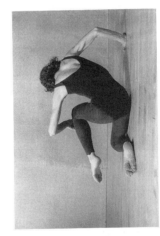

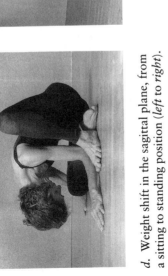

d. Weight shift in the sagittal plane, from a sitting to standing position (*left* to *right*).

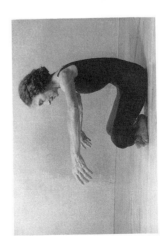

e. Weight shift in the horizontal plane, involving rotation (*left* to *right*). Variation on work with Erick Hawkins.

103

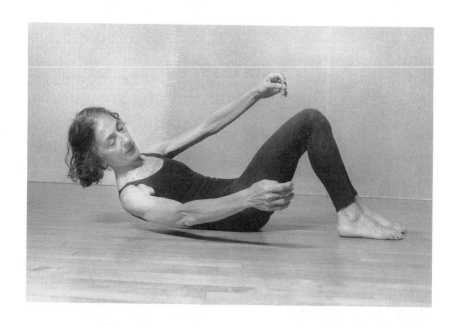

f. Abdominal strengthening. Karipides engages her abdominal muscles in an isometric contraction (*above*). An advanced form of this exercise is shown (*below*), in which the weight of the legs is used for resistance.

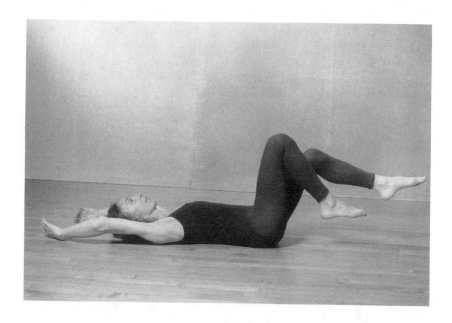

also believes that body parts must work in opposition to each other: as one limb flexes, the other extends.

The work emphasizes weight shifts initiated from the center of gravity rather than the upper torso or extremities (Figs. 27b–f). This is true of much work in modern dance. What distinguishes Karipides' sequence of movements is her emphasis on feeling anchored to the floor as well as feeling anchored internally. The work is actually a folding and extending of the extremities with the "sit" bones (ischial tuberosities) as anchors.

Karipides begins her strengthening session by contracting the abdominals upon exhalation, folding or shaping the torso. This movement is a preparation, a patterning for all other strengthening work. The emphasis is on dynamic movement using full range of motion rather than on isometric exercise.

In all of Karipides' work, the strengthening comes from the constant use of the torso muscles to maintain dynamic alignment. There is no progressively heavy overload included in her program. Thus, she will be able to maintain her strength, but not increase it. This is no problem for Karipides—she is stronger than most dancers half her age. *Critical to maintaining her strength is the fact that she performs her regimen every day, whether she is sick, healthy, busy or not.*

Much of Karipides' "body work" is also found in the technique classes she teaches. She urges all dancers to find personal "body work" that effectively meets their own training and performance needs. With the technical demands of dance (arguably) increasing and dancers continuing to dance in their forties and beyond, finding a personal maintenance and conditioning regimen is essential. The regimen must be compiled not from "tradition" or what "feels good," but from what serves best to meet personal health and professional goals.

Karipides' movement exercises are presented in progression: "rolling," "rocking" in different planes (front and back, side-to-side), weight shifts in different planes, and abdominal strengthening, followed by movement exercises at the stall bars.

"ROLLING" SIDE-TO-SIDE, FRONT-AND-BACK (**Fig. 27a**). It is only Karipides' strong pelvic muscles that prevent her from bruising bony extensions of her body. She often begins her movement sequence with rolling after a warm-up such as walking or light running in place.

FRONT-AND-BACK (SAGITTAL PLANE) "ROCKING" (**Fig. 27b**): KNEES EXTENDED AND THEN FLEXED. In performing this movement, it is important to feel a sense of "abandon." This is possible only if the abdominal muscles are sufficiently strong to help stabilize the torso—allowing for a "scooped," "hollow" feeling—rather than relaxed (allowing the stomach to bulge). The arms and legs are free to move as long as the muscles that stabilize the lower spine are sufficiently strong.

TWISTING SIDE-TO-SIDE AROUND THE VERTICAL AXIS (**Fig. 27c**). The arms fling, but control of the torso is maintained. This movement exercise and the one shown in Figure 27b can be taxing to the cardiovascular system.

WEIGHT SHIFT SEQUENCE IN THE SAGITTAL PLANE, FROM A SITTING TO A STANDING POSITION (**Fig. 27d**). During this sequence, careful attention must be paid to the alignment of the ankle, knee, and hip joints. Initiation is from the center of gravity—the pelvis—with each change of position.

WEIGHT SHIFT SEQUENCE IN THE HORIZONTAL PLANE (INVOLVING ROTATION) (**Fig. 27e**). From a sitting position, the movement is initiated with a contraction. The body rotates to one side, abdominal muscles working throughout the movement. The contraction of those muscles initiates the return to the sitting position.

ABDOMINAL STRENGTHENING (**Fig. 27f**). Karipides uses her abdominal muscles in an isometric contraction, with both shoulder blades off the floor. The stomach is "scooping" rather than "bulging." Karipides is strong enough to isolate the deep abdominal muscles.

An advanced form of this exercise is also shown, in which the abdominals are constantly engaged, the back is pressed to the floor, but the weight of the legs is used for resistance. The hip flexors are neutralized by maintaining the legs with the knees at a 90-degree angle. Care must be taken not to hyperextend the lower back and not to flex the hip so that the knee is directly in line with the hip joint; the knee should be moved away from the hip joint so that the abdominal muscles work throughout the entire exercise. Note that the cervical spine should be as relaxed as possible. Karipides usually incorporates this exercise into a longer movement sequence: eight counts to lift the

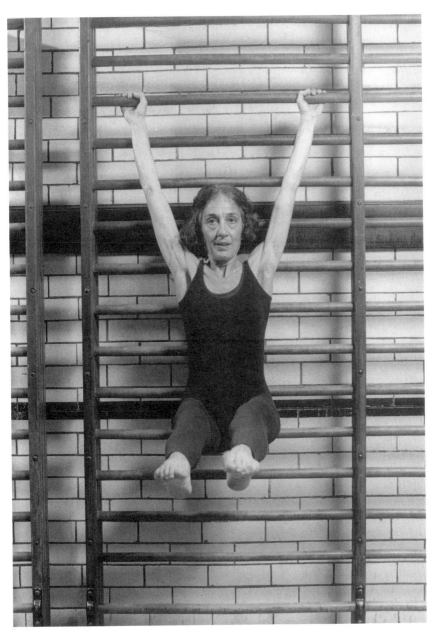

Figure 28. Strengthening the hip flexors using stall bars. *(Photo by Mike Sands)*

legs off the floor; four counts to lower; two to slide the legs along the floor; four to slide the legs back along the floor and return to the starting position.

STRETCHING AND STRENGTHENING USING THE STALL BARS (**Figs. 8a, 28**). In Figure 8a, Karipides assumes a stride position, stretching the inner thigh muscles and at the same time strengthening her shoulder girdle and upper back musculature to lift herself above the floor. Lower-back and abdominal musculature is also working. In Figure 28, she strengthens the hip flexors.

Much of the strengthening work illustrated here will result in tightening of the hip flexors if the abdominal muscles are not sufficiently strong to support the body. Hip flexor tightness and weakness (e.g., psoas insufficiency syndrome) results in stretched and weakened abdominal muscles, which restricts turnout at the hip, and causes other compensations.[7]

HIP FLEXOR STRETCH USING THE STALL BARS (**Fig. 29**). This exercise alleviates hip flexor tightness. It can be performed with the back leg turned in or turned out. Full stretch is achieved with the leading foot slightly in front of the knee. Note also that Karipides is "pressing" her hips to the floor.

Strength Training Using Increased Resistance

Dancers are generally aware of the importance of strong abdominal muscles, but safe movement of the torso is also facilitated by, for example, strong back muscles. Also, the invariably weaker hamstrings and lower-leg muscles usually need strengthening. Considerable lower-back pain and malalignment of the lower body joints can occur if these muscles are weak and/or tight.

Dancers thus need to work all their major muscle groups with increased resistance and increased variation in the workout to realize fitness gains. Increased resistance is important because over time specific bodily adaptations to a given amount of resistance will occur. The body adapts *exactly* to what is demanded of it; unless the demand or stress placed on the body is increased and varied, there will be no increase in strength.

A General Adaptation Syndrome (GAS), first described by Dr. Hans Selye, provides a framework with which a strengthening program using overload can be designed for dancers.[8] The basic

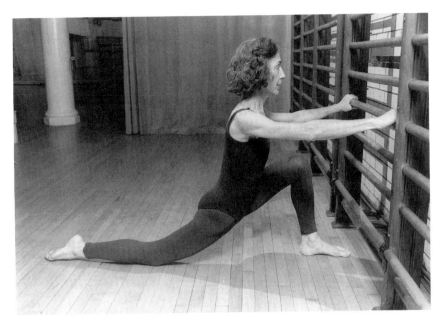

Figure 29. Hip flexor stretch using the stall bars. *(Photo by Mike Sands)*

theory states that whenever any stressor (e.g., exercise, disease) is experienced by the body, adaptations are made (after an initial response of shock or alarm) so that future exposures to the stressor will be less disruptive. Over time, a strenuous workout program results in specific and quantifiable as well as nonspecific bodily adaptations.[9]

Thus, strength-training programs should:

- begin gradually to ease through the shock or alarm phase of GAS
- be varied in content, intensity, and duration of workouts for optimal improvement
- include occasional breaks from the routine to change the stressor input to the body and to avoid damage to the tissues.

Exhaustion and injury may result if a program is not carefully constructed.

Karen Clippinger-Robertson points out:

Overload criteria indicate the importance of careful class design to provide the appropriate magnitude and progression of overload. If class demands are too similar from day to day, there will be insufficient overload for the desired improvement. [On the other hand, dance] teachers and students . . . are notorious for noticing a weakness or problem and wanting it changed immediately. . . . This approach utilizes too extreme an overload applied for too short a time. . . . Careful selection of an appropriate mode of progressively increasing overload in small increments over several months is often necessary to achieve the desired gains.[10]

In addition to overload, specificity is important in designing training programs. Optimal gains may require a training overload similar in intensity and duration to the goal movement. For example, performing slow tendus has little relation to building the strength needed for fast grand battements; many of the same muscles are used, but the velocity and hip joint angle are quite different and there is different recruitment of muscle fiber types.[11]

The principles given above can easily be applied to a strengthening program in dance:

- The easier workout may begin with two sets of ten repetitions (reps), moving to three sets of six reps, and eventually to three sets of ten reps.
- The number of reps performed in the program, however, should vary with the movement exercise. For example, the larger muscle groups should be worked fewer reps than the abdominals and smaller or single muscle groups.
- High reps (above fifteen) to fatigue should be avoided if strength development as opposed to muscular endurance is the goal.

However, correct technique in lifting should never be sacrificed for higher resistance (lifting more weight). Even a minimal hiking of the hip when lifting the leg to the side can have a dramatic effect on the way the muscles are used. *Correct technique in lifting includes appropriate breathing patterns—inhale just before starting the more strenuous phase of the movement, and exhale as the movement is completed. The dancer should control the movement through its full range, rather than rely on the momentum of the movement.[12] This does not mean that the movement always has to be performed slowly.*

The speed of the movement is part of the intensity component of a training program. The speed with which the movement exercises are executed affects the way the body adapts to them. If the muscle groups being exercised are used "explosively" in the movement the dancer is training for, such as large jumps, then the specific movement exercise should be performed quickly. This also assists in neuromuscular learning—training the nervous system. In addition, it helps to prepare the tendons and other connective tissue to withstand the large forces and accelerations required in the jump.

Usually, when it becomes possible to lift the current resistance for a greater number of repetitions in the set, the resistance must be increased. This does not mean that the weight must be increased consistently; on a three-day-per-week program it would be best to have one heavy, one light, and one medium training day. Remember that some type of variability must be incorporated into any training program if progress is to result. Runners, for example, run different distances at different paces (intensity) from day to day. Otherwise, total adaptation of the body occurs and there is no event sufficiently specific to result in strength gains.

Larger muscles should be exercised first because smaller muscles tend to fatigue more readily. For example, if the goal is to develop leg and hip strength, leg presses (Fig. 30a) and other lower-body exercises should be performed first. The rest of the movement exercises should be put in a specific order so that single-joint movement exercises (Figs. 30c–h and 31b–d) come last.

Above all, the individual needs of the dancer must be considered in designing any conditioning program. Exercises that closely replicate movement demands of the dance form should be used. It is clear that many dancers are not interested in bodybuilding and muscle definition per se. Rather, they are more concerned with the strength increments needed for the repertory or movement they are dancing, which may vary throughout the season.

In view of their functional needs, dancers should actually train in cycles: strength training for a given period of weeks (this can also be done between rehearsals); followed by stamina and general fitness conditioning, perhaps preparing mentally and emotionally by reading, looking at videotapes of other performances, or talking with coaches. This is referred to as periodization of training.[13]

APPLICATIONS: SAMPLE PROGRAM USING ELASTIC BANDS

There are a number of elastic bands commercially available for conditioning programs. The resistance is usually determined by the thickness of the band. Bands of different thicknesses can be used individually or in combination for greater resistance.

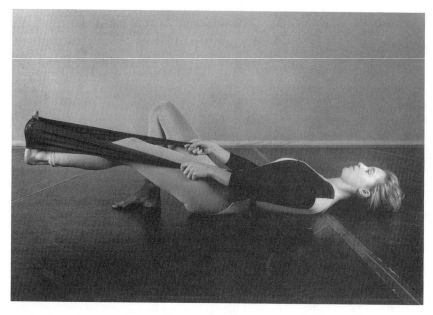

a. Quadriceps and lower leg strengthening.

Figure 30. Judy Gantz's strengthening regimen using Therabands. *(Photos by Anthony Hall)*

Precautions should be taken when doing resistance work with the bands:

- Trainees with hypertension problems should be especially careful in performing high-resistance work; they should consult a physician before starting a conditioning program.
- Trainees with a history of knee problems should perform abduction and adduction movement exercises with the band tied above the knee joint.
- All exercises should be performed through the full range of motion of the joint.
- In standing exercises especially, correct alignment must be maintained at all times.
- Trainees should breathe evenly while performing the exercises, exhaling on the exertion phase of the movement.[14]

Using the regimen of dance kinesiologist Judy Gantz, illustrated in Figures 30*a–i*, the elastic bands can be used to strengthen the upper-body shoulder and back muscles, as well as the large muscle

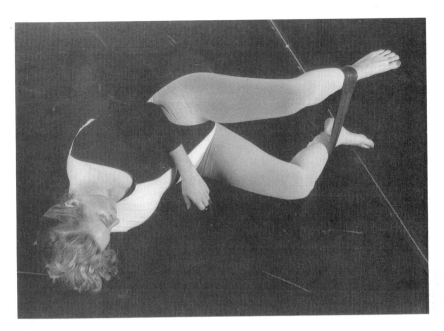

b. Hip abductor and lateral hip rotators strengthening.

groups of the lower body. The pattern of resistance should match the pattern of resistance demanded in dance. For example, the hip extension action in Figure 30*f* is similar to that needed for an arabesque.

All of the strengthening movement exercises in Figure 30 should be performed in three sets of ten reps for three days a week.[15] The intensity—the amount of resistance worked against the band—should be varied for strength gains to occur: one day should be heavy, one medium, and one light. Dancers should start slowly with the exercises before pushing for heavier resistance work loads.

Quadriceps and lower leg strengthening (Fig. 30*a*). Lying supine (face upward), place the band around the foot, holding one end of the band in each hand. In this and all exercises with the band, the band must be held tightly so that it does not snap back. Starting with the knee bent to the chest, press the leg slowly until it is straight—completely extended along the floor. Return to the starting position and repeat.

Hip abductor and lateral hip rotators strengthening (Fig. 30*b*). Lying on the back with the knees bent, tie and place the band above both ankles. Slowly pull the legs apart while turning out at the hip joint.

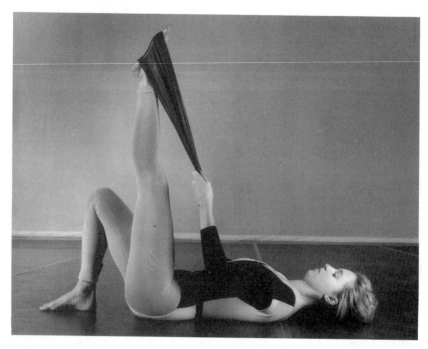

c. Calf strengthening.

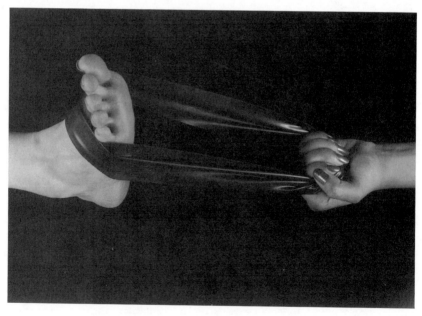

d. Front lower leg (ankle dorsiflexors) strengthening.

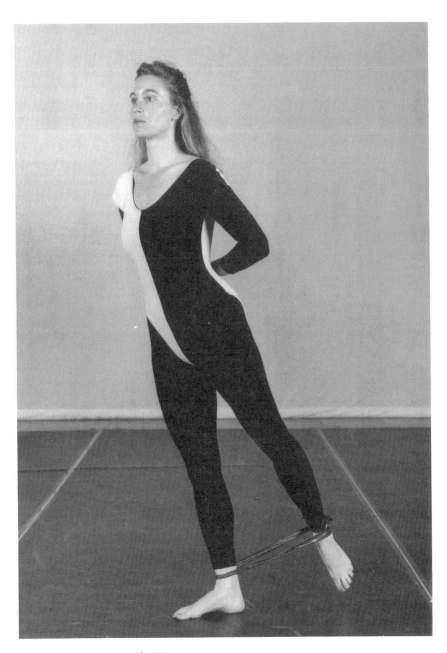

e. Hip extension strengthening.

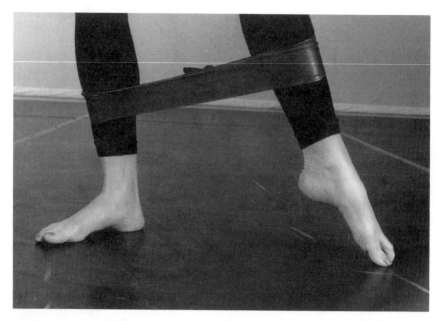

f. Hip abductor strengthening.

Keep the lower back securely on the floor, being careful not to arch it. Feel the muscles working on the side and back surfaces of the thigh and buttocks.

Calf strengthening (Fig. 30c). Lying supine, place the band around the foot, holding one end of the band in each hand. Slowly point the foot, working against the resistance of the band. Dorsiflex the foot to recuperate and repeat.

Front lower leg (ankle dorsiflexors) strengthening (Fig. 30d). Place the band around the midfoot area, with a partner holding it. Dorsiflex the foot, drawing it back toward the shin. Feel the muscles working on the front of the lower leg.

Hip extension strengthening (Fig. 30e). Place the tied band around the lower leg/ankle area. Starting from a turned-out first position, slowly reach the leg backward, working the muscles along the back of the thigh and the buttocks area.

Hip abductor strengthening (Fig. 30f). Tie the band with a secure knot around the lower legs and from a turned-out first position, slowly move the leg sideways in a tendu, feeling the resistance along the outside of the thigh. Return to the starting position and repeat.

Hip adductor strengthening (Fig. 30g). Standing in a turned-out

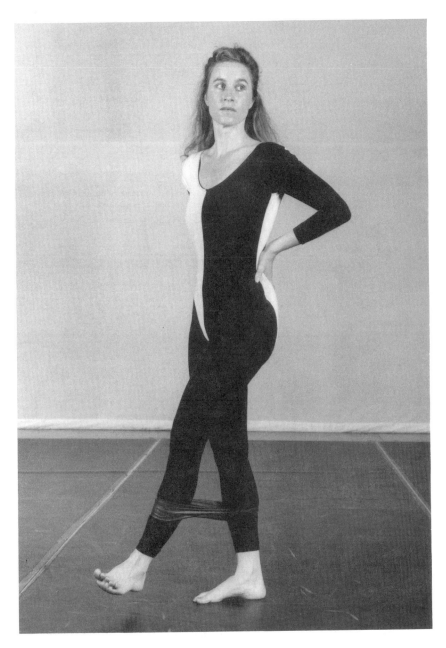

g. Hip adductor strengthening.

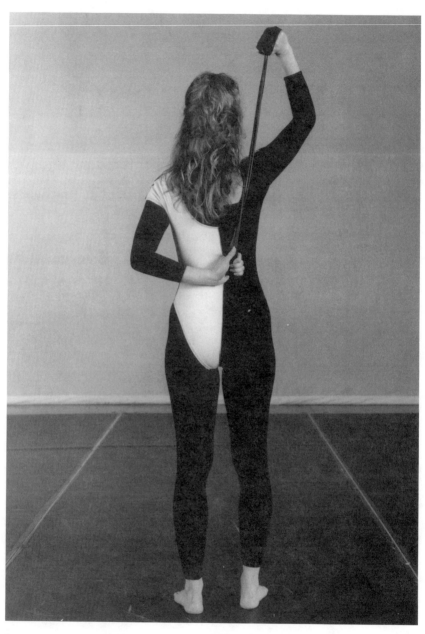

h. Upper arm strengthening.

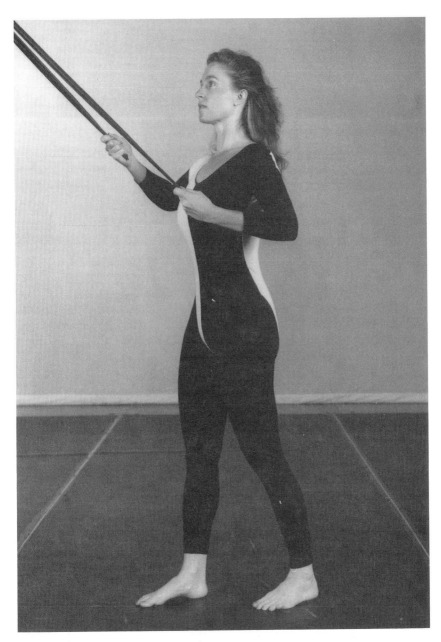

i. Back and front lower arm (latissimus dorsi, posterior deltoid, elbow flexors) strengthening.

position, knees relatively straight, with the band tied and placed around the lower legs, pull one leg across and in front of the standing leg. Feel the muscles working on the inner thigh.

Upper arm strengthening (Fig. 30*h*). Standing, holding one end of the band in one hand behind the back, place the other end of the band in the other hand, both elbows bent. As the arms straighten, one arm extends toward the ceiling. Alternate arms. Feel the muscles working along the back side of the upper arm.

Back and front lower arm (latissimus dorsi, posterior deltoid, elbow flexors) strengthening (Fig. 30*i*). The band must be secured around a hook or held by a partner. Standing with the feet apart and facing forward, one end of the band held in each hand, reach arms straight forward. The band is slowly pulled down and backward, while the elbows are allowed to bend. Return to starting position and repeat. Abdominals should be engaged during the pull to avoid arching the lower back.

APPLICATIONS: SAMPLE PROGRAM USING MACHINES

Companies such as Universal, Nautilus, Cybex, and Eagle produce resistance machines for strengthening work. The machines are easy to use—resistance is adjusted merely by changing the position of a metal pin. Compared to free weights, machines are often preferred in large facilities because of their convenience and their safety features.[16] A sample strengthening program using Cybex machines is given below.[17]

Dancers are often exposed to Cybex machines in rehabilitation. Cybex research specialist and former dancer Robin Chmelar works with dancers, instructing them in the use of the Cybex and Eagle machines for injury treatment and general conditioning. Chmelar says that "Cybex training is great for rehabilitation because it provides for training at high speeds, up to 300 degrees per second, which is very important for dancers whose joints need to function at high speeds."[18]

Illustrations of some strengthening movements that Chmelar prescribes are given in Figures 31*a–h*. Like most dance movement specialists, Chmelar also believes that trunk extension and flexion are an essential part of *any* strength-training program:

> Jumping and arabesque [movements] require tremendous strength in the trunk extensors, not only to execute the movement but also to stabilize the spine. I find many dancers fear strengthening their extensors thinking they will become lordotic

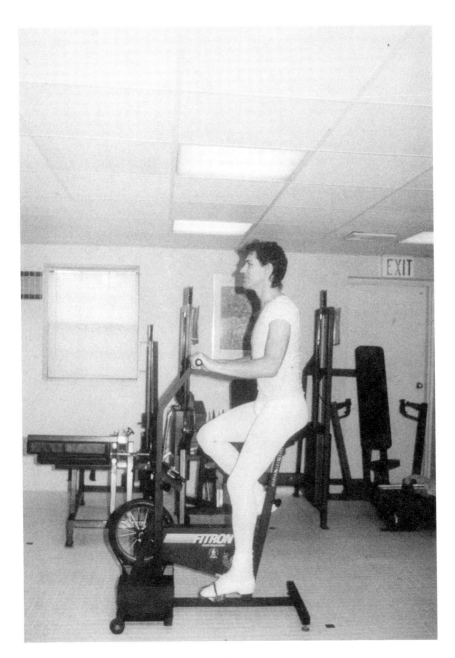

a. Strengthening work must be preceded by a warm-up.

Figure 31. Jerel Hilding, formerly of the Joffrey Ballet, shows strengthening exercises using Cybex machines. *(Photos by Robin Chmelar)*

(hyperextended). This is a misconception and consequently many dancers end up in a vicious cycle of back injury and extensor weakness that never gets addressed. The abdominals are important, too, but dancers should pay particular attention to the rotation component—with greater emphasis on the obliques and not just on the rectus.[19]

The specific trunk extension and flexion exercises that Chmelar recommends, included in the following descriptions, are not performed on a Cybex machine; rather, hand weights can be used for added resistance.

To begin this and all strengthening programs, it is important to warmup. Figure 31*a* shows former Joffrey Ballet dancer, Jerel Hilding, in a pre–weight training warm-up. He is cycling at about 90 rpm on the Cybex Fitron Isokinetic Ergometer. For dancers with patellofemoral problems, the seat height should be adjusted so that the knee is in no more than 15 to 20 degrees of flexion. An "aerobic" workout can also be performed on the same machine (i.e., for a longer duration of twenty to sixty minutes) for cardiovascular training.

The following movement exercises should be performed in three sets of ten reps. The frequency should be three days a week. Note that the plate weight and cam resistance[20] vary widely among manufacturers. The guidelines given below apply only to Cybex equipment.

QUADRICEPS STRENGTHENING (**Fig. 31*b***).
Equipment: Cybex Leg Extension.
Weight (plates): 12.5 lbs/plate. Goal is 75 percent of body weight in pounds, but the initial level may be as low as one plate.
Resistance: Variable according to the cam system, ranging from 7 to 11 pounds. To set for individual needs, the number of plates should be sufficient to fatigue by the tenth rep, but not so much that three sets of ten cannot be completed.
Rest: Thirty seconds between sets.
Variations:
1. To stress the eccentric component of the movement, raise the bar with both legs but lower with only one. Set the resistance only to eccentric tolerance to prevent muscle soreness.
2. To emphasize muscular endurance, increase reps to fifteen and decrease resistance by approximately one-third of the ten-rep maximum or to tolerance.
3. To emphasize muscular strength, decrease reps to five and

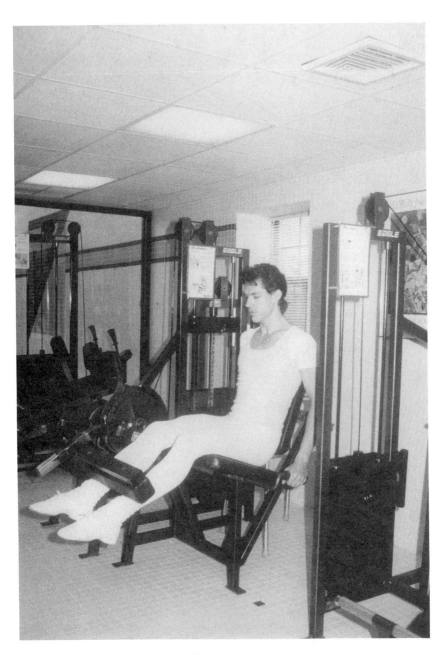

b. Quadriceps strengthening.

increase the resistance by approximately one-third of the 10-rep maximum or to tolerance.

4. Dancers with patellofemoral problems may use the range-limiting device so that the extension motion starts at anywhere from 45 degrees (mid-range) to 20 degrees of flexion. This reduces the compressive forces on the patella.

HAMSTRINGS (AND GASTROCNEMIUS) STRENGTHENING (**Fig. 31c**).
Equipment: Cybex Leg Curl.
Weight (plates): 12.5 lbs/plate. Goal is 50 percent of body weight in pounds, but the initial level may be as low as one plate.
Resistance: Same as for Cybex Leg Extension.
Rest: Thirty seconds between sets.
Variations: Same as for Cybex Leg Extension 1.–3.

GASTROCNEMIUS (AND ACHILLES TENDON) STRENGTHENING (**Fig. 31d**).
Equipment: Angle Board (or Slant Board).
Duration: After warm-up, hold twenty to thirty seconds and release. Repeat.

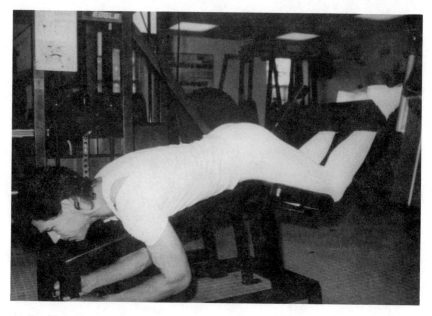

c. Hamstrings (and gastrocnemius) strengthening.

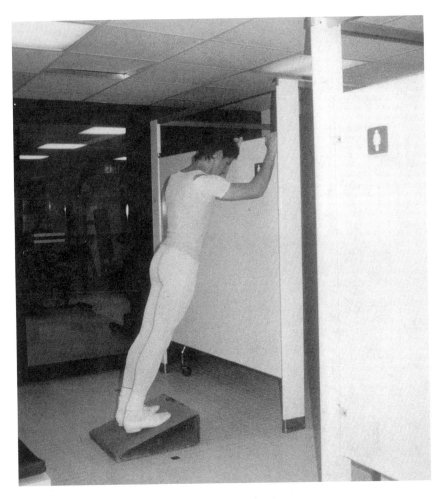

d. Gastrocnemius (and Achilles tendon) strengthening.

Sets: Three to five.
Frequency: Three to five days a week.
Variations:
1. Internally rotate the hips so that the toes point inward to enhance the stretch to the lateral head of the gastrocnemius.
2. Flex the knees slightly in parallel position to stretch the soleus.

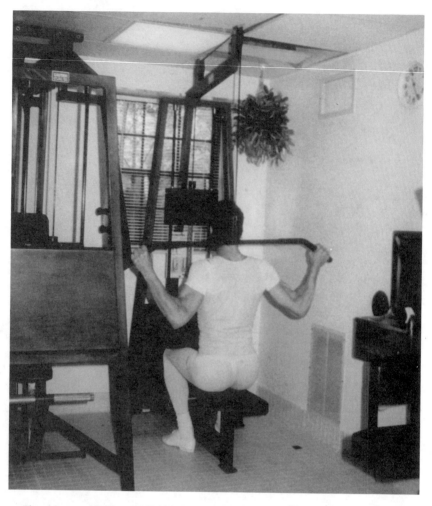

e. Shoulder or glenohumeral adductors, scapular downward rotators, and elbow flexors strengthening.

SHOULDER OR GLENOHUMERAL ADDUCTORS, SCAPULAR DOWNWARD ROTATORS, AND ELBOW FLEXORS STRENGTHENING (Fig. 31*e*).

Equipment: Cybex Lat Pulldown.

Weight (plates): 12.5 lbs/plate.

Resistance: There is no set goal. Since the bar weighs 10 pounds, one plate is equal to only 2.5 pounds of resistance.

Rest: Thirty seconds between sets.

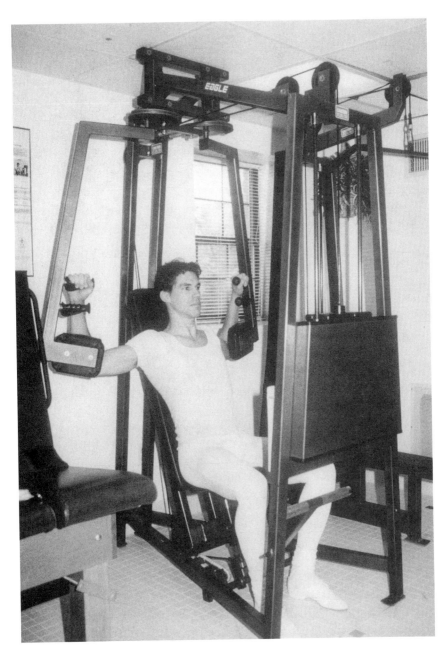

f. Glenohumeral horizontal adductors—pectoralis major, anterior deltoid, coracobrachialis, biceps (short head) strengthening.

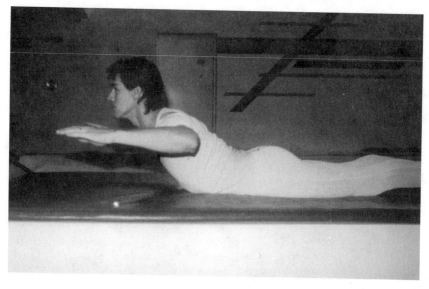

g. Trunk extensor (muscles of the scapula) strengthening.

Variation: The bar may be lowered, alternating posterior (as in the Figure) with anterior pull. The posterior pull emphasizes the scapular muscles; the anterior pull emphasizes the pectorals.

GLENOHUMERAL HORIZONTAL ADDUCTORS: PECTORALIS MAJOR, ANTERIOR DELTOID, CORACOBRACHIALIS, BICEPS (SHORT HEAD) STRENGTHENING (**Fig. 31*f***).
Equipment: Cybex Fly Machine.
Weight (plates): 12.5 lbs/plate.
Resistance: There is no set goal.
Rest: Thirty seconds between sets.
Note: The pectorals should be stretched following this exercise.

TRUNK EXTENSOR (MUSCLES OF THE SCAPULA) STRENGTHENING (**Fig. 31*g***).
Resistance: The resistance varies with the arm position. For greater resistance, the arms can be raised overhead. For less, the arms should be positioned along the side of the body. Hand weights may also be added.
Duration: Ten reps, hold each rep for a count of ten (the arms should provide enough resistance so that the tenth rep is almost at the point of muscle fatigue).

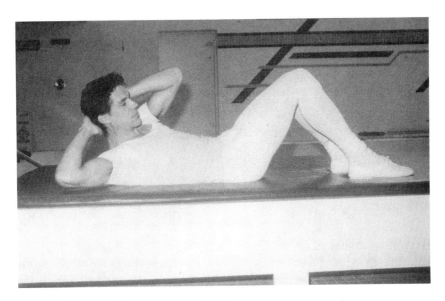

h. Trunk flexors and rotators strengthening.

Rest: Thirty seconds between sets.
Variations:
1. Extend the spine and rotate, alternating reps right and left.
2. Extend and laterally flex, alternating reps right and left.
3. Extend the torso over the edge of the mat table so that the torso is hanging forward in flexion, as in the beginning position.

Note: The legs may or may not be stabilized by a partner. Also, postinjury, the degree of hyperextension should be gradually increased according to tolerance. This exercise should be followed by static stretching, both for lumbar hyperextension and flexion.

TRUNK FLEXORS AND ROTATORS STRENGTHENING (**Fig. 31***h*).
Resistance: The resistance varies with the arm position. For greater resistance, the arms can be raised overhead. For less, cross the arms over the chest. Hand weights may also be added.
Duration: Ten reps, hold each rep for a count of ten (the arms should provide enough resistance so that the tenth rep is almost at the point of muscle fatigue).
Rest: Thirty seconds between sets.
Note: In this exercise, the torso lifts off the floor only to the thoracic spine; the body does *not* curl up to the knees. This is to avoid

pressure on the intervertebral discs and to concentrate the action on the abdominal muscles, rather than the hip flexors.

APPLICATIONS: PILATES

Pilates technique has been used by dance pioneers such as Ruth St. Denis, Ted Shawn, Martha Graham, Helen Tamiris, Hanya Holm, Pearl Primus, and George Balanchine. It is one of the most common methods of strength training used by professional dancers today.[21]

Originally, the conditioning work consisted of a series of exercises performed on a mat. Later, Joseph Pilates designed the "Universal Reformer," a sliding horizontal bed on which the dancer may pull or push against a metal bar or leather straps. The resistance is provided by detachable springs. Many dance movements, such as plié, relevé, développé, and battement, can be performed in turned out and parallel positions with the machine. Other parts of the program feature abdominal work (for which many dancers use Pilates technique unassisted by machines). Pilates is also useful in rehabilitative work, since much of it is performed in a non-weight-bearing (non-standing) position. Two selected examples of Pilates exercises are given below.

One problem with the Pilates technique is that much of it is performed in hip flexion. Dancers who train with Pilates machines and exercises may develop tight hip flexors. They must make sure that the strengthening work is followed by systematic stretching of the hip flexors such as shown in Figure 32 (this stretch can also be performed with the foot of the front leg flat on the floor, as in Figure 29).

Hip flexors strengthening.   Lying supine on the "Universal Reformer," with a leather strap added for resistance (the strap is attached at the head of the horizontal bed and around the feet), flex the hips to approximately 45 degrees. Return to the starting position and repeat.

Triceps strengthening.   In relevé, reach behind and hold onto the equipment handles, slightly hyperextend the shoulder and spine and lift the body away from the machine. The abdominals are also strengthened as they support the lower back.

APPLICATIONS: SAMPLE PROGRAM USING FREE WEIGHTS

Free weights are often recommended for strength training in dance because they require dancers to balance both themselves and the weight, rather than allow the machine to do it. This results in greater muscle coordination during the exertion phase of a movement.

Free weights also permit a freer range of movement; machines are more limiting in this respect. Some machines have great two-dimensional range of movement, but they do not imitate freely moving bodies accelerating in three-dimensional space.

Muscle groups are not worked in isolation in dance. Thus, a sample strengthening program should emphasize multiple-joint exercises. These are often called "total body" exercises since many joints and muscles of the body are involved.[22] Two examples are given.

Push jerk: hip and leg extension (explosive strength or power). This exercise begins with hand-held weights resting partly on the shoulders. Bend the knees, then thrust the weights straight upward with quick knee and hip extension. Lastly, the weights are caught and held steady overhead with the knees bent, which straighten for final support.[23]

Lunge: hip and leg extension. This exercise can be performed with either hand-held dumbbells or a barbell held on the shoulders behind the head. With the dumbbells, grip strength is also developed, especially as the load is increased.

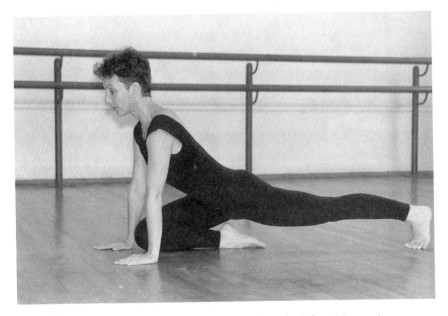

Figure 32. Cathy Paine in a hip flexor stretch. *(Photo by Julyen Norman)*

The movement begins from a parallel standing position; vertical alignment is maintained throughout by isometric contraction of the spinal erectors. Move one leg forward in a lunge and lower the body to the floor so that the lead knee is approximately over the lead foot at the lowest part of the lunge. Reverse the movement by pushing up and back with the lead foot. It may take several small backward steps to return to the original parallel position.

Alternate legs. Advanced trainees can perform five to ten consecutive lunges on the same leg before alternating sides. For dancers, it is probably best to alternate legs to avoid fatiguing the muscle.

As a variation, the barbell can be held on the front of the shoulders and clavicles. Also, the movement can be completed by stepping forward rather than back.

As with all exercises with free weights—barbells and dumbbells—dancers must be very careful to maintain good vertical alignment throughout the movement, especially when increasing the intensity of the workout (heavy weights or higher reps).

As more and more professional companies offer weight-training facilities and dancers are able to afford the time and money to work in private studios and gyms, dancers will become more comfortable with using free weights. Bruce Marks, artistic director of the Boston Ballet, says:

> Weight training in professional ballet is no longer the exception, it is the norm. Our new studios will have a strength training room complete with Pilates and Universal machines, barbells, and dumbbells. Dancers need to train with the free weights, especially to meet the demands of the abstract and modern ballets in our repertory.[24]

Endurance

Physiologically, dancers often resemble strength athletes. In one study, the morphology of the heart—the left ventricle's muscular wall—was similar to that seen in athletes trained for strength.[25]

Much of dance takes place in intervals of several minutes followed by varying periods of rest. The movement is either moderately intense with a strong isometric component during adagio dancing or it is a highly intense, brief-duration exercise, such as jumps or leaps (Figs. 33a–b). Sometimes this highly intense exercise must be sustained. In the original staging of *Annie Get Your Gun*, Daniel

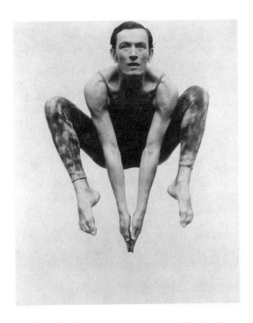

a. Don Redlich in performance. *(Photo by John Lindquist)*

Figure 33. Dance is characterized by short-burst activities such as jumps and leaps.

Nagrin was required to run and jump for two-and-a-half minutes with one four-second break, ending with sixteen continuous jumps in place, twelve of them split-jumps.

Dance movements can thus be categorized according to the length of work and the power required. The movements listed in Table 4 would not be considered true "endurance work"—at least fifteen to twenty minutes in which the dancer maintains a heart rate of 60 to 80 percent of maximal heart rate.[26]

The heart rates of dancers during performances of classic ballets such as *Swan Lake* and *La Bayadère* have been measured by researchers.[27] They found that the longest single period of nonstop dancing was seven minutes and that the overall performance demands tended to fall into the category of interval work: two to three minutes of intense activity followed by two to three minutes of rest. For such work, dancers primarily use immediate/short-term energy systems. Energy must be generated very rapidly, usually in an oxygen-free (anaerobic) muscular environment. Even if oxygen were available, it could not be used fast enough to be of much use in the production of energy.

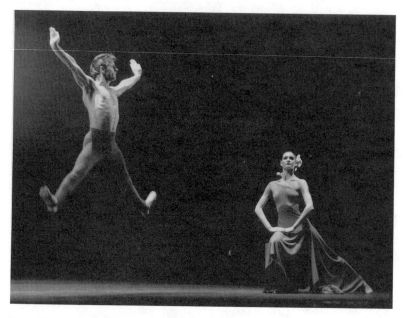

b. Mikhail Baryshnikov with Maxine Sherman. *(Photo by Jed Downhill)*

To train the short-term energy system, activities must be selected that engage the muscles needed for power movements. This usually involves strength training that increases the intensity of overload during maximum bursts of effort.

Table 4. Duration and Power Requirements of Dance Movements

Exercise	Duration	Power
Tendu en croix	30 secs.	Moderate intensity
Rond de jambe with allegro component	60 secs.	Moderate intensity
Combination with "swings"	30 secs.	Maximum short-burst
Combination with jumps	30 secs.	Maximum short-burst

Although most dance cannot be characterized as true, uninterrupted endurance exercise, continuous movement performed for more than two minutes—as in Nagrin's solo mentioned above—will use energy from aerobic as well as anaerobic energy systems. This work requires dancers to have a highly trained oxygen transport or aerobic energy system and a well-conditioned heart and vascular system that can circulate large quantities of oxygenated blood for relatively long durations. The weak link in oxygen delivery (unless one has a respiratory disability) is the cardiovascular, not the pulmonary system. Dancers also usually try to maintain low body fat, and endurance work may be essential to fat breakdown.[28] Throughout the remainder of this chapter, "endurance" will refer to cardiovascular, not muscular, endurance.

Dancers must be able to sustain physical activity with little fatigue, especially since fatigue is an important factor in the causation of injury. In training and rehearsal, dancers become easily fatigued when, for example, their technique is incorrect (e.g., sickling the foot in relevé) or inadequate (e.g., landing from a jump without loading weight on the heel); when they have not had enough fluid (i.e., at least 64 ounces per day) or carbohydrate intake (see Chapter 5); and when they are stressed or overloaded with training and performance commitments.

Fatigue is a way of life for many professional dancers. They must cope with it and, more importantly, learn to minimize it. One way to do this is to condition the heart and blood vessels for efficient delivery of oxygen to the working muscles, thus reducing muscular fatigue— pain resulting from a high rate of accumulation of lactic acid, which is responsible for stimulation of nerve endings located around muscle fibers and also interferes with muscle contraction and regeneration of the muscles' energy-producing material (ATP, or adenosine triphosphate).

Much of the movement Twyla Tharp choreographs could be classified as endurance exercise. The rehearsals should have almost a training effect for the dancers, especially when the company runs two demanding pieces, *Sue's Leg* and *Four Down Under*, back to back. Much of the choreography of Margalit Marshall (Fig. 34) and others—Lucinda Childs, Laura Dean, Molissa Fenley, Danny Smith/ Joanie Shapiro—is also "aerobic." It is continuous, moderate exercise for at least twelve to fifteen minutes.

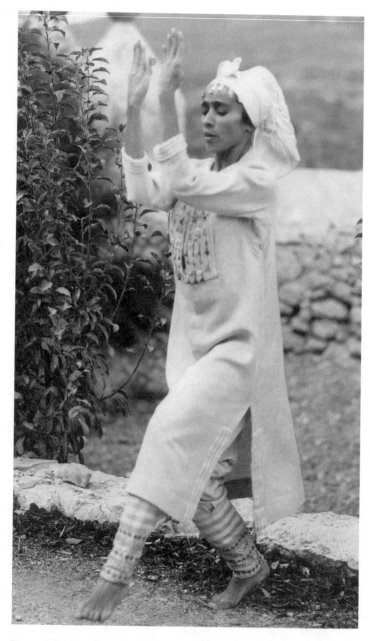

Figure 34. Margalit Marshall in performance. *(Photo courtesy of Margalit Marshall)*

Endurance Conditioning

REHEARSAL

What training do dancers receive to be able to dance at a moderate intensity uninterrupted for fifteen minutes or more? Often the training is the rehearsal. As researchers Steven Chatfield and William Byrnes suggest, advanced and professional dancers—without any supplemental training—seem to have above average aerobic capacities when compared with the general population (20 to 30 milliliters/kilogram/minute [ml/kg/min]).[29] Their review of the literature is presented in Table 5.

According to Chatfield and Byrnes, using rehearsals of the performance for conditioning guarantees the specificity—if not the overload—needed for increments in endurance. The energy systems involved in the performance will be targeted in the training as will the specific muscles and reflex patterns used for the performance:

> First, imagine a twenty-minute piece that requires all dancers to be on-stage for the entire time. [The] steps [elicit] a steady state heart rate near 160 beats per minute. . . . In the second piece there are two contrasting dynamics: One is explosive, utilizing jumps, leaps, kicks, lifts, and throws which elicit heart rates of up to 200 beats per minute for 30 to 45 seconds; the contrasting dynamic lasts 60 to 135 seconds and is a smooth, calm series of sustained, stationary, slow motion gestures allowing the dancers' heart

Table 5. Aerobic Capacity of Dancers

VO_2max^a of Dancers in the Study	ml/kg/min
Beginning dance students	31^b
American Ballet Theatre	44, 48 (women, men)^c
Royal Swedish Ballet	51, 57 (women, men)^d

[a]VO_2max is the maximum amount of oxygen that an individual can utilize to produce energy required for work. It is expressed in units of milliliters of oxygen per kilogram of body weight per minute (ml/kg/min) and is considered an acceptable measure of the ability of the cardiovascular system to deliver oxygen to the working muscle. Typical values for sedentary individuals range from 20 to 30 ml/kg/min.

[b]From J. A. DeGuzman, "Dance as a contributor to cardiovascular fitness and alteration of body composition," *Journal of Physical Education and Recreation* 50 (1979): 88–91.

[c]From J. L. Cohen, K. R. Segal, I. Witriol, and W. D. McArdle, "Cardiorespiratory responses to ballet exercise and the VO_2max of elite ballet dancers," *Medicine and Science in Sports and Exercise* 14 (1982): 212–217.

[d]From P. G. Schantz and P. O. Astrand, "Physiological characteristics of classical ballet," *Medicine and Science in Sports and Exercise* 16 (1984): 472–476.

rates to recover to below 100 beats per minute. These two dynamics continually alternate throughout the piece. The cardiovascular demands of these two pieces are antithetical. Rehearsing for one piece would not condition a dancer to perform in the other.[30]

SUPPLEMENTAL AEROBIC TRAINING

The concept of training specificity describes how measures of performance are specific to training modes. For example, if a piece of choreography requires a dancer to run for two minutes, drop to the floor, return to standing, and jump backward for thirty seconds, the best way to train for the requisite endurance is to rehearse the specific movement.

However, supplemental training can also be beneficial to improvement of the dancer's overall endurance.[31] For example, adding swimming to dance training can "improve overall endurance [and] offer the physiological and aesthetic benefits of breathing with less labor during performance. . . . [In addition, the swimming adds] very little risk of musculoskeletal injury during the supplemental training."[32]

Certainly, the time demands of dance training limit how much exercise outside of dance can be done. In terms of priorities, strength training and flexibility need to be emphasized in conditioning programs for dancers. Nevertheless, to the extent that the training does not interfere with the dancer's timing or cause injury (e.g., when jogging "toed-out"), endurance exercise should be encouraged in dance training. Exercising three days per week for at least fifteen to twenty minutes is a good starting regimen in a conditioning program.

To vary the program, the frequency (from three to five days), duration (up to forty or more minutes depending on the intensity), and intensity (up to 80 to 85 percent of maximal heart rate) can be increased. These components are considered separately below. Whatever the aerobic activity chosen for the program, it must provide an adequate overload to the heart and vascular system, and it must develop the aerobic capacity of the specific muscles that are worked—usually the larger leg muscles.

It is not *continual* progression, but *varied* progression that is important in conditioning. Dancers are not training to run marathons but to increase stamina in class and performance. Progress need not be immediate, but rather slow and steady. This is especially important, given the time constraints on dancers. Most dancers aren't able to squeeze daily thirty-minute workouts into their training schedules.

Frequency. Of the three training components, *frequency guidelines are the least flexible. The trainee must work out at least three times a week.* However, the good news is that "more is not necessarily better"—exercising five or six days a week does not necessarily produce greater cardiovascular gains than exercising three days a week. The gains depend more on the intensity and duration of the exercise.

This is not to say that if dancers have time to work out only one or two days a week that it is not worth the effort; an extra day or two might eventually be worked into the busy schedule. Above all, it is very important for dancers to feel that this is not just "something else" that must be added to their already overfilled training regimen. Likewise, if dancers want to exercise five or six days a week, although increments in cardiovascular fitness (relative to working out three or four days a week) may not be seen, the calorie expenditure resulting from the exercise may be worth the time commitment.

Duration. There is some debate over this component. If fifteen minutes is good, is forty-five minutes better? Not necessarily. Bouts of short, moderate exercise might help to promote fitness; studies have shown that three ten-minute jogging workouts a day, five days a week for eight weeks (at moderate intensity) increased the aerobic capacity of participants.[33] Fit individuals who run approximately one mile as fast as possible four days a week will require only about thirty to forty-five minutes of total exercise time per week. The fitness gains, however, may be dramatic owing to the intensity of the exercise.

Clearly, the exercise does not have to be long-duration to show fitness gains. Nevertheless, dancers must be very careful if they engage in high-intensity/high-impact endurance activities such as running or jogging. Injury might result if they have any structural or muscular imbalance (e.g., patellofemoral problems or muscular imbalance of the hip rotators).

Intensity. Some published studies indicate that high-intensity exercise—exercising at high target heart rates—results in better fitness gains and higher caloric expenditure if it is intermittent.[34] Previously, it was thought that exercise must be continuous in order to show a training effect (i.e., the heart muscle must be subjected to continual stress and not allowed to "relax" during the training bout).

However, intermittent exercise—alternating high-intensity movement with moderate- or low-intensity work—may result in greater fitness gains.

Another interesting finding comes from a fitness study of healthy men and women that appeared in the November 1989 issue of the *Journal of the American Medical Association*.[35] Ever since its publication, dozens of newsletters and magazines have reported that people don't have to be marathoners to greatly improve their fitness level. The study found that of the five groups of people categorized according to fitness levels, the least-fit group derived the largest benefits from moderate exercise—walking briskly for thirty to sixty minutes every day.

Few dancers would qualify for inclusion in the least-fit group of study participants. Nevertheless, future studies will probably show that *for individuals at a moderate cardiovascular fitness level, moderate-duration and moderate-intensity exercise is effective in realizing fitness gains. What does this mean for dancers? Walking on a regular basis is probably the best exercise.* Cycling and swimming should also be considered.

SOME CONSIDERATIONS IN SELECTING TRAINING MODES

Running. Dancers should be careful in selecting weight-bearing endurance exercise. Their muscles must be sufficiently strong to support the exercise (e.g., for running, the inward hip rotators must be strong enough to prevent "toeing-out," a cause of injury).[36] Dancers can check for this by imagining a line that runs down their chest and extends between the legs and the feet. As they run, their feet should be on each side of and parallel to the line—*not* toed-out. In addition, proper athletic shoes that provide shock absorption, flexibility, and support must be worn.

Cycling. Dancers often fear that they will develop "big thigh muscles" by cycling. This is true if they cycle with heavy resistance. To concentrate on cardiovascular conditioning rather than muscle strengthening, they need cycle only with light resistance applied (see section on strength training). Dancers with patellofemoral problems should cycle with no more than 15 to 20 degrees of knee flexion.

Swimming. It may be that swimming "works the wrong muscles for dance" in terms of balancing the strength of all the large muscle groups or that relatively higher body fat percentages are maintained by swimming compared with other aerobic training activities. However, these problems are unlikely for dancers, who swim at low-intensity levels. Many dancers enjoy the recreational as well as conditioning aspects of the sport. It is particularly useful for rehabilitation when there has been an injury to the lower body and weight-bearing exercise is contraindicated. Movements that might stress the lower back muscles (e.g., the butterfly stroke) should be performed only when supporting musculature is sufficiently strong.

Walking. With hand weights or without, walking is safe and enjoyable endurance exercise. Compared with other aerobic training modes, it is certainly easier on the knees and lower body joints—especially if there are no steep inclines to walk down (deceleration can irritate some of the connective tissue in the knee). A number of studies have shown that substantial caloric expenditure can be achieved with certain walking regimens. This low-intensity exercise—for long durations—will demand a large percentage of its "fuel" as fat rather than as glycogen or "stored" carbohydrate; thus, there are implications for fat management.

Nonimpact aerobics. Dancers should also consider nonimpact aerobics for endurance training as well as for developing creativity and expressivity. This exercise combines numerous movement forms and rhythms with various visualization techniques. Shoes need not be worn. Training heart rates are achieved by frequent changes of level and continuous, active use of the upper body. This technique should not be used by individuals with knee or shoulder disabilities.[37]

Other indoor and outdoor training modes. There are other forms of endurance exercise (jumping rope, chair stepping, canoeing, cross-country skiing, and so on) that could be included in a program. There are also other factors in the fitness program to consider, such as training to condition a particular muscle-fiber type.[38]

Assuming that dancers don't have the time to stroll for two hours in the local foothills or city park, or strap on the cross-country skis, find some snow, and go touring for forty minutes, what would a cardiovascular conditioning program for dancers look like? Dance researchers Robin Chmelar and Sally Fitt offer an answer. They have combined the principles discussed above into some very workable exercise guidelines.

For example, Week One/Day One to Two starts off with fifteen minutes of exercise (all of which should be low-impact or non-weight-bearing (e.g., walking, cycling, swimming) in intervals of three minutes at 60 percent of the maximal heart rate and two minutes at 70 percent. The interval set is thus five minutes, which is repeated three times for a total fifteen-minute workout. Two minutes are added for the seventeen-minute bout on Day Three. As the fitness level increases, the workouts gradually become longer. The program includes variations in frequency, duration, and intensity.[39] Each exercise bout should be preceded by a warm-up and concluded with a "cool-down" that is essentially the reverse of the warm-up, resulting in a gradual decrease in body temperature.

Flexibility

Flexibility is defined as the range of motion around a joint or set of joints. Researchers speak of both static and functional flexibility. *Static flexibility* is the range of movement produced statically without using the momentum of the movement itself. Of particular interest to dancers is *functional flexibility*, the ability to move a joint with little resistance during actual dance movements. Flexibility is usually achieved through stretching, a specific form of exercise designed to increase or maintain flexibility.

For functional flexibility, much is required of dancers in terms of strength and neuromuscular coordination. For example, to perform a side leg extension (Fig. 35), sufficient strength is needed to raise the large weight of the leg. The timing of external rotation of the hip (engaging the deep outward rotators to "drop" the hip under effectively) and extension of the knee (raising the knee high before beginning to straighten the leg) are also very important to achieve the desired height.[40]

Traditionally, stretching exercises have been purported to be a necessary part of a warm-up and injury-prevention program in dance and sports. However, one warms up to stretch, not the other way around (see Chapter 3). There is also some confusion about the relationship between flexibility and injury prevention. Beyond moderate flexibility, there is probably no further injury-prevention effect offered. Extreme flexibility may be associated with higher risk of injury to connective tissues, especially if muscle and structural imbalances and other risk factors are present.[41]

A more significant benefit of flexibility is its influence on technique (to avoid the pathogenic compensations that dancers make when structural limitations restrict flexibility) and on muscle properties. Certain mechanical properties of muscle, such as peak-force development and speed of contraction, may be enhanced by rigorous stretching—although not so rigorous that muscle cross-bridges are permanently broken—potentially enhancing speed and

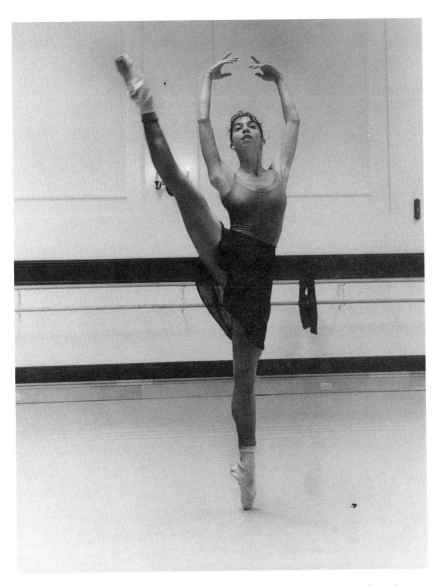

Figure 35. Valerie Madonia performing a leg extension to the side. *(Photo by Weiferd Watts)*

efficiency during performance.[42] Stretching can also increase proprioceptivity (i.e., the ability of neural system components to sense position and placement) and serve as a biofeedback mechanism to reduce pre- and postperformance stress.[43]

Much of the resistance to flexibility is individual and genetic in nature; therefore, flexibility should be approached on an individual basis. Stretching techniques themselves are part of a dynamic pedagogy, changing constantly.

Ever since Herbert A. De Vries published his paper on static stretching (see Bibliography) in 1962, this mode has been widely used in technique classes of all dance idioms. Research now shows that proprioceptive neuromuscular facilitation (PNF), which involves a contract/relax procedure, probably yields the greatest increases in flexibility over time. These gains, however, may not be long-lasting.[44]

Stretching Techniques

What limits flexibility? The greatest resistance to stretch comes from the fascial sheath (a sheath of connective tissue support) that covers the muscle.[45] Certainly, the dancers' skeletal physical limitations, emotional state, and ability to relax as well as environmental factors such as room temperature will also influence the range of flexibility. In general, the joint capsule and articulations account for about 47 percent of flexibility, tendons and ligaments about 10 percent, muscles and fascial sheaths about 40 percent, and skin about 2 percent. It is the muscles, fascial sheaths, and skin that should be emphasized in any stretching technique, *not* the relatively inelastic connective tissue.

STATIC STRETCHING, also known as stretch-and-hold, is a low-force, long-duration method. Usually the position is held anywhere from thirty to sixty seconds. In the stretch, the muscle is held in a position of elongation greater than its resting length. There should be a stretching sensation, but no pain.

SLOW STRETCHING involves a gradual lengthening of a muscle group, but the stretch is never held. When the muscle is in a maximally stretched state, it is then released. This can become a more "static" technique if the terminal position is sustained. In teaching stretch classes, I personally prefer to combine slow stretching with static methods for certain muscle groups, in particular, the hamstrings.

BALLISTIC STRETCHING depends on the speed and weight (momentum) of the moving body part to lengthen the muscle. An example of a ballistic hamstring stretch would be a leg swing from a back lunge position to the front and return to the starting position, with repeats. The problem with ballistic stretching is that the force generated from the fast stretch to lengthen the muscle operates against a protective (stretch) reflex contraction of the same muscle group. This combination of opposing forces may result in muscle tears and injury. However, ballistic stretching may be as effective as static methods for increasing flexibility.[46]

PNF STRETCHING is derived from a clinical rehabilitative program and has since been applied to dancers and other athletes in training.[47] This method of stretching usually requires a partner.

The method involves placing the muscle group (e.g., hamstrings) to be stretched in an elongated position; gradually contracting the muscle group isometrically until a near-maximum effort is obtained (e.g., in a supine position, lowering the leg to the floor against resistance provided by a partner [Fig. 36] or an elastic band); sustaining the contraction for four to ten seconds, followed by relaxation of the muscle group;[48] returning the leg to the beginning position, then stretching it (i.e., static stretch of the muscle for thirty to sixty seconds).[49]

The only problems with PNF techniques are that the person assisting with the stretch must be well informed about the technique and the correct alignment that must be maintained throughout the stretch (watching especially for "cheating" during the contraction phase), and that this method takes considerable time, especially in a class situation.

In addition to static, ballistic, and PNF techniques, stretching can also be categorized according to who or what is responsible for the range of motion. In *passive stretching*, the motion is performed by a partner or special equipment (e.g., traction). In *active stretching*, the motion is accomplished solely by the activities of one's muscles; there is no outside resistance or assistance.

Relying mainly on passive stretching is not advised because the dancer will develop mainly passive flexibility—this is not very useful in performance. Dancers must also be careful when using passive stretching to avoid extreme and rapid stretch, possibly activating the stretch reflex.[50]

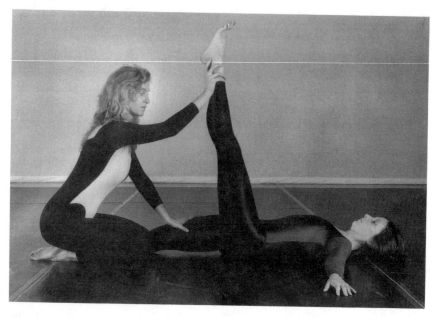

Figure 36. PNF (proprioceptive neuromuscular facilitation) technique is used to increase the flexibility of the hip joint and the elasticity of the hamstrings. *(Photo by Anthony Hall)*

Stretching Programs

GENERAL PRINCIPLES
Some general principles apply to all methods of stretching:

- Flexibility training sessions should be preceded by a warm-up of at least five to fifteen minutes, whatever is needed to increase the body temperature 1 or 2 degrees.
- It is especially important for dancers to be relaxed, since the ability to reduce muscle fire (i.e., to relax certain muscles so that others are able to stretch or activate) is critical to successful stretching.
- Effective stretching requires a relatively quiet environment, a passive attitude, relaxed breathing, and a reasonably comfortable position.
- Exercises can be performed with the eyes closed, to help concentration and visualization of the correct performance of the exercise.
- Frequency and duration of the stretching program must be

varied so progressive adaptations result. (The *routine* stretching in ballet class—not to mention other dance forms—is hardly sufficient to result in any improvements in flexibility.)

- Stretching three times a week is probably adequate to maintain flexibility. The less flexible dancer should try to stretch at least five times per week. Dancers with particularly tight muscle groups should stretch several times a day—especially after class when the muscles are warmer and more pliable.

Duration refers not only to the length of each session and number of stretching exercises used, but also to the length of the hold phase of the static (thirty to sixty seconds) and PNF methods. It may be difficult for beginning students to sustain a stretch for more than ten seconds without "pulsing" or "bouncing," in which case monitoring the time and giving verbal cues may help.

There are many warnings that dance researchers, educators, physical therapists, and kinesiologists give to dancers regarding stretch programs. Perhaps none are so cogent or vociferous as those given by Judy Alter: *do not bounce, lock (hyperextend), arch the lower back or neck, swing, do fast exercises, or "overbend" a joint.*[51] These can be expanded:[52]

1. Do not hyperflex the knee or neck.
2. Do not hyperextend the knee, lower back, or neck.
3. Do not apply a twisting force to the knee (see discussion of torques in Chapter 3).
4. Avoid holding the breath (on inhalation) during the stretching exercise.
5. Avoid overstretching any joint so that the ligaments and joint capsules are stretched.
6. Avoid passive neck stretches.
7. Avoid stretches that place acute compressional forces on spinal discs, such as extending and rotating the spine simultaneously.

QUESTIONABLE EXERCISES

There are a number of stretching exercises that are questionable and should be avoided or modified:[53]

- Stretches using excessive flexion of the lumbar spine (e.g., in a standing hamstring stretch, leaning over as if touching one's toes with unsupported lumbar flexion; back muscles relax, leaving the unsupported ligaments and vertebral discs of the spine to support the weight).

- Stretches using excessive hyperextension of the lower back and cervical spine (e.g., as in a back-arching abdominal stretch, possibly causing impingement on the nerve, compression, and even herniation of the disc and myofascial trigger points).
- The yoga "plough" (the dancer is supine with the legs extended over the head, feet touching the floor; this is inappropriate because of the large compressive forces placed on the cervical spine).
- The hurdler's stretch (the rear foot is usually flared out to the side, placing stress on the medial aspect of the knee and overstretching the medial ligaments, not to mention causing increased strain on the lower back).

Some stretches are useless rather than dangerous, often because there are "weak links" in the "stretching chain" to prevent the desired muscle group from stretching. For example, tight hamstrings (the "weak link") may prevent a dancer from actually feeling a stretch in the lower back musculature, or the reverse.

Given that many of these exercises are questionable, dancers may still be asked by choreographers to perform some of the movements. What should dancers do? First, determine whether or not the movement is actually risky, then decide whether or not to perform the choreography. If the decision is to perform, dancers can then begin to condition the body to be able—at least partially—to withstand some of the stresses that the movement places on the body. This conditioning emphasizes strengthening (e.g., neck and upper back musculature for many jazz movements) and training to maintain good alignment (e.g., of the upper torso joints), but can also include some flexibility work (shoulder and shoulder girdle muscles).

It is important to remember that many of the exercises considered dangerous do not allow for individual differences. In a clinical setting, in which the correct execution of the movements is supervised, some of these "dangerous" exercises—especially when modified—may actually be quite useful.[54] Two examples are the prone quads stretch (Fig. 37a) and the modified hurdler's stretch (Fig. 37b).

In the prone quads stretch, proper alignment of the knee and hip joints is maintained by the dancer holding onto the foot with both

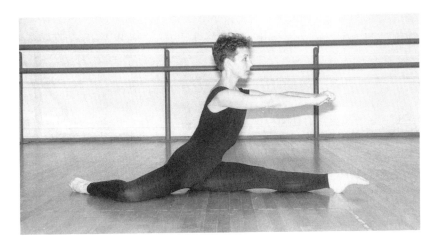

a. Prone quads stretch.

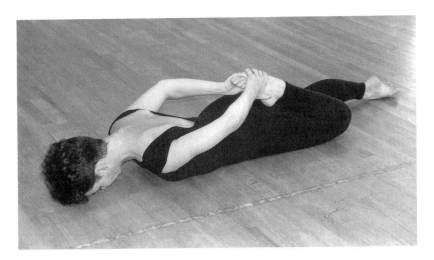

b. Modified hurdler's stretch.

Figure 37. Modifying potentially hazardous stretching exercises. *(Photos by Julyen Norman)*

hands as opposed to just one. The stretch can be increased by allowing the thigh to come off the floor, taking care not to pull down on the foot and hyperflex the knee. In the modified hurdler's stretch, the rear foot is not allowed to flare to the side, which would result in overstretched medial ligaments. By pressing forward, increased strain on the lower back is avoided.[55]

EXERCISES BY DANCERS AND FOR DANCERS

Robert Stephens, director of sports medicine and associate professor of anatomy at the University of Health Sciences in Kansas City, Missouri, was a leading dancer in Ballet Midwest for more than ten years. He has since developed a comprehensive injury-prevention program.[56]

The program features strengthening exercises that are followed by stretching exercises in the following sequence: abdominals/back, internal/external rotators of the hip, hamstrings/quadriceps, superficial/deep calf, plantar flexors/dorsiflexors of the ankle. They consist of slow, progressive static stretches, held for thirty to sixty seconds, and contract/relax or PNF stretching. The PNF stretches are especially effective for the hamstrings, groin muscles, and quadriceps. Stephens emphasizes the importance of breathing, relaxing, and visualizing to facilitate the slow and correct performance of the exercises.[57]

Karen Clippinger-Robertson, a former dancer who studied with Bill Evans and Kelly Holt, is a kinesiologist for Seattle Sports Medicine and a consultant to Pacific Northwest Ballet and the U.S. Weightlifting Federation. She has designed a flexibility program that is especially useful for beginning dancers and dancers with rather limited flexibility.[58]

These dancers must concentrate especially on stretching the chest and upper body musculature, the hip flexors, external hip rotators, groin muscles, hamstrings, hip abductors and iliotibial band, and deep and superficial calf muscles. The program emphasizes all of these muscle groups. Clippinger-Robertson has published another series of exercises for dancers, some of which use PNF principles unassisted by a partner.[59]

Two other excellent sources of specific stretching exercises are Judy Alter's books (see Bibliography), which emphasize *safe* stretching. Simply and clearly described, they are recommended for casual exercisers as well as dancers. The more flexible dancer may need to modify some of the stretches using PNF techniques.

As with all exercise regimens—and flexibility programs are no exception—the dancer must vary exercise/training components if increases in flexibility are to be made. For flexibility work, this usually means increasing the duration or the frequency of the session, or the intensity (perhaps by using different stretches), until acceptable flexibility is achieved and can be maintained.

Profiles

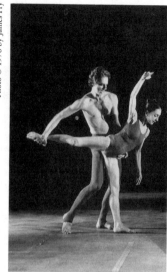

Kathryn Karipides

An indefatigable teacher, dancer, and performer, Kathryn Karipides co-chairs with Kelly Holt the dance program in the Department of Theatre Arts at Case Western Reserve University in Cleveland, Ohio. From 1969 to 1979, she was the co-director, choreographer, and principal dancer for the Dance Theatre of Kathryn Karipides and Henry Kurth. In that ten-year period, the company gave approximately 100 performances. Compared with modern dance companies that have one or two "seasons" (e.g., in New York) and touring commitments, an average of ten performances a year might seem like a "light" schedule. Karipides continues to perform two or three times a year. She has no intention of quitting, perhaps because she monitors her workload so carefully.

Now in her mid-fifties, she boasts that she has never suffered an injury in dance—her only musculoskeletal injury was a medial meniscus tear from a moped accident in 1980. She gives credit to her training in Danish gymnastics and in dance (with Hanya Holm, Martha Graham, Erick Hawkins, and study abroad at the Mary Wigman school in West Berlin, the Laban Art of Movement Studio in England, and the Dalcroze Institute in Switzerland) for her long and healthy performing career.

Each day she gives herself a class based on "fundamental movement principles" and strengthening exercises (described on pages 101–108). This one-hour workout helps her to maintain innate strength and stamina. How long will she continue to dance? Karipides smiles.

> I have spent so many years learning and maturing, why should I throw it all away now, just when I'm working at my best? My range of movement may have decreased some, but my line and length are still there. I'll stop dancing when the preparation for performance becomes agonizingly painful or long, when the joy in the preparation and the doing is no longer there, when it becomes a chore. [Full] maturity as a performing artist doesn't ever happen until a dancer reaches his or her late thirties and early forties. With this maturity comes an intelligence that tells you how to work best.

It's an intelligence that serves her well.

• • • • • • • • • • • • • • • •

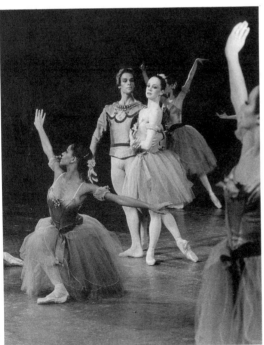

Photo courtesy © Steven Caras, 1990

Daniel Duell

Unlike most professional dancers, Duell's interests have always extended beyond the studio and the stage. For ten years he served as the NYCB representative to the American Guild of Musical Artists (see discussion of AGMA in Chapter 6). He also served as a guest lecturer for NYCB Guild seminars and educational programs, "to enhance the public's understanding of ballet and to develop new audiences for ballet." His interests are wide-ranging—he is also an accomplished classical musician—but much of the critical acclaim he receives has been for his dancing.

Duell began studying ballet at age eleven. At age twenty, he was invited to join NYCB. Five years later he advanced to the rank of soloist and after two years was promoted to principal dancer. He has danced leading roles in Balanchine's *Coppélia, Harlequinade, Agon, Symphony in C, Donizetti Variations, Stars and Stripes,* and *The Four Temperaments.* He has also danced principal roles in Jerome Robbins's ballets, including *The Goldberg Variations* and *Dances at a Gathering.*

Many of these roles were what Duell calls "hard jumping roles." Now, as artistic director of Ballet Chicago, he continues to perform on occasion, but principally teaches and choreographs. He began choreographing in 1980 with his *3 Preludes,* set to the music of George Gershwin. Most of his works now are choreographed for and danced by Ballet Chicago, for which he wants to develop a "dynamic, forward-looking repertoire."

Duell is especially concerned about the technical training of his company. He says that dancers must be trained to dance without conscious effort, "to move instinctively without calculation."

> Men especially need to be very careful in lifting partners. This usually means they need some strength training or rehabilitative weight lifting. This is not for muscle definition. Rather, it is to help align the body, to place the arms and shoulders to full mechanical advantage. There are basic principles of weight management in the air that must be learned, and the men must be strong enough to use them. Especially in partnering, the technique of the dancers, or lack thereof, really shows.

Duell encourages the dancers he directs at Ballet Chicago to lift free weights: "Every dance studio ideally should have accessory exercises and systems." Duell also incorporates alignment, strength, and breathing exercises based on yoga principles into the company's training regimen. For so many years he worked on giving compelling performances; now he helps others to do the same.

· · · · · · · · · · · · · · · · · ·

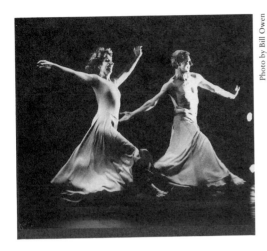

Photo by Bill Owen

Kelly Holt

Kelly Holt began dance training at age fifteen at the University of Georgia, where he earned a B.F.A. in Theatre Arts. Directing civic and military theatrical productions for four years in the U.S. Air Force eventually brought him to New York. Holt was to enjoy fifteen more years of study, performing, and teaching in New York before taking a university position. In New York, he danced with Erick Hawkins (an affiliation that lasted over ten years), the Herbert Berghof Studio, the Theatre of the Open Eye, Dialogue House, and New York University's Tisch School of the Arts.

Although he continues to perform, it is in his role of teacher that he feels most comfortable. He currently co-directs the graduate dance training program at Case Western Reserve University in Cleveland, Ohio. In the summer, he teaches at the Summer Dance Theatre Institute at the University of California, Santa Cruz.

His approach to technique and correction is not one of blind dedication, but of inquiry. Always asking, "What more can I learn?" he has tried many therapies and treatments. Recently, he has undergone a course of Rolfing.

The commitment to inquiry has served him well. He has sustained no injuries in dance and has continued to dance well into his fifties. He attributes this to his way of working. Always having struggled with a limited range of motion, he spends a disproportionate amount of time stretching.

More important than stretching in his training is involvement of the psyche with the physical aspects of dance. The opportunities for exploration of the mind-body relationship are endless when one rejects the "sweat-and-shower" approach to training. As a teacher, Holt is committed to a holistic educational approach:

> [It provides] technical know-how that involves reliably effective training in the psychological processes underlying the phenomenology of creativity, an atmosphere of energized investigation. . . . A place where students and faculty are looking for appropriately contemporary and serviceably fulfilling answers within the depths of themselves and within the living dynamic of their ongoing development.[60]

He believes his approach to self-involving contemporary training, drawing heavily but not exclusively on principles inherent in Hawkins's approach to dance training, is "liberating and animating."

• • • • • • • • • • • • • • • • •

Photo courtesy of Monnaie Dance Group/Mark Morris

Keith Sabado

It was a fateful day in 1974 when Keith Sabado gave up his premedical studies for a liberal arts course of study in the humanities.

He has since studied with many notable figures in contemporary dance—Hannah Kahn, May O'Donnell, Alvin Ailey—and become a danseur noble of modern dance. But it is his association with Mark Morris that has brought the most rewards—financial* and artistic. It has also been mutually beneficial for the two artists; some critics refer to Sabado as Morris's "muse." This is perhaps an overstatement, but it is true that Sabado is a stunning dancer and figures prominently in much of Morris's work.

Although he enjoys being asked by Morris "to do things that he never thought possible," Sabado tries not to throw himself into a piece, although that's what usually happens. When he's not careful, injuries result—recurring shoulder spasm, lower back pain, sprained and inflamed ankles, stress fractures in the metatarsal joints, muscle strains in the lower leg. With each injury, there is a knowledge that comes from the pain. Most of that knowledge comes to him when he is quietly lying on the floor, "trying to figure things out."

Sabado is a devotee of Pilates work and considers it essential for strengthening his muscles and preventing further injuries. Even so, the injuries come, "but you have to find the balance between the physical and the emotional, the pain and the excitement of performing." By all critical accounts, this dancer in his mid-thirties has done just that. With or without injuries, he will continue to dance "until age forty and beyond, as long as the desire is there."

*In September 1988 Mark Morris brought his company by invitation to Brussels as the Monnaie Dance Group/Mark Morris. At the time of this interview, Sabado repeatedly mentioned the move to Belgium. It represented something of an anomaly in dance: a full-time salary and adequate benefits.

———— Five ————

Nutrition and Diet

Dancers are concerned about nutrition; many are obsessed by it. In general, dancers eat too much of certain nutrients—too much protein, too much fat—while depriving the body of much-needed carbohydrates.[1] Some have chronic eating disorders,[2] while others have a daily energy consumption far below the Recommended Dietary Allowances (RDA) of 1,900 to 3,000 Calories or kilocalories* (see Table 6). The major source of calories in the diet should be high-carbohydrate foods that also provide protein.

Researcher Jane Bonbright has calculated that approximately 15 kcal/lb/day (kilocalories per pound of body weight per day) is needed for the body to function under normal circumstances.[3] Dancers must add another 200 to 300 kcal/lb/day to meet class, rehearsal, and performance energy demands. Many dancers' energy consumption, however, is even lower than their basal metabolic needs—the minimum amount of energy needed to sustain the body's vital functions. The resting or basal metabolic needs usually represent about 60 to 75 percent of the RDA.

Nutrient imbalances, especially of calcium, are also a problem among dancers. This is particularly true for women. Postmenopausal and amenorrheic dancers produce less estrogen and, especially those

---

*A calorie is a unit of energy; a Calorie or kilocalorie equals 1,000 calories. Throughout this chapter, Calories and kilocalories will be used interchangeably.

Table 6. Summary of Caloric Intake Among Adolescent and Adult Dancers[a]

Study	Population	Daily Calorie Intake Mean (Range)
Bonbright (1989)[b]	female students— professional schools (Washington, D.C.)	1,584 (642–2,611)
Benson et al. (1985)	female students— professional schools (California)	1,890 (700–3,000)
Clarkson et al. (1985)	female students— professional schools (Massachusetts)	1,776 (784–2,513)
White (1982)	female adults—Ballet West (Utah)	1,282 (722—2,043)
Calabrese et al. (1983)	female adults— Cleveland Ballet (Ohio)	1,358 (550–2,115)
Cohen et al. (1985)	female adults— American Ballet Theatre (New York)	1,673 (977–2,361)
Hamilton et al. (1986)	female adults—four national ballet companies (United States)	1,894 (650–3,758)
Cohen et al. (1985)	male adults—American Ballet Theatre (New York)	2,967 (1,739–4,104)

[a]Some of these data have appeared in tabular form in Robin Chmelar and Sally Fitt, *Dancing at Your Peak: Diet* (Princeton, N.J.: Princeton Book Co., Publishers, 1990). Note that the range in energy Recommended Dietary Allowances (RDA) for females is 1,900–2,200 kcal and for males is 2,300–3,000 kcal.
[b]The entries for references in this table can be found in the Bibliography. See also E. Bright-See et al., "Nutrition beliefs and practices of ballet students," *Journal of the Canadian Dietetic Association* 39 /4 (1978): 324–331; A.P. Kvasova, "Evaluation of a balanced diet for students at a ballet school," *Higiena Sanitariya* 8 (1974): 27–29.

with a dietary history of calcium deficiency, are at high risk for osteoporosis (adult bone loss in which the bone becomes porous). Osteoporosis begins early in life and progressively worsens with prolonged calcium deficiency. (Dietary sources of calcium are given in Table 8.) A woman's bone loss at age thirty-five is already twice that of a man's at age fifty. Exercise may help to slow the rate of bone mass loss. Many dancers take mineral and vitamin supplements, but these are neither complete nor balanced. Bonbright has found that although 33 percent of her study group used nutritional supplements, only 15.6 percent used a complete and balanced vitamin/mineral supplement, with nineteen essential vitamins and minerals supplying 100 to 150 percent of the RDA.[4]

Energy Nutrients: A Primer

CARBOHYDRATES

Carbohydrates contain carbon, hydrogen, and oxygen in a specific ratio of two hydrogens for each oxygen. They are categorized as monosaccharides, a six-carbon sugar group such as glucose, fructose, and galactose; disaccharides, consisting of two simple sugar molecules, such as glucose and fructose, to form sucrose; and polysaccharides, consisting of three or more simple sugar molecules, most commonly cellulose, starch, and glycogen.

All carbohydrates, whether in the disaccharide or polysaccharide form, must eventually break down in digestion into glucose for energy metabolism.[5] A small amount may be stored as glycogen, and those carbohydrates that are resistant to human digestive enzymes are excreted from the body. Besides serving as the body's primary energy nutrient (and usually the only energy source for the central nervous system), glucose facilitates the complete breakdown of fat. Each gram of carbohydrate provides about 4 kcal.

The monosaccharides and disaccharides are together referred to as simple sugars. Foods containing some of these sugars are, for example, brown sugar, corn syrup, honey, and white grape juice. Excessive amounts of any simple sugar can result in body fluids being drawn quickly into the intestinal tract, together with a decrease in blood glucose levels. There is evidence that certain sugary foods that are high in fat, such as ice cream, release glucose over a relatively long period of time, similar to some polysaccharides.

Cellulose and polysaccharides such as pectin make up the fibrous parts of plants and are thus sources of "dietary fiber." They are common in leaves, roots, seeds, and other plant structures.

A single starch unit can consist of thousands of sugars strung together, such as in breads and other grains, beans, and potatoes. These foods are referred to as "complex carbohydrates."

Glycogen is a polysaccharide of particular importance in energy management. It is usually found stored in the liver, where it is transformed from glucose in a process called "glycogenesis." It is also found in the muscles, totaling an average reserve of up to 3 percent of muscle cell weight (less than 1 pound). When glucose is needed to maintain blood glucose levels, liver glycogen is reconverted to glucose in a process called "glycogenolysis." This glucose is then available for use by the working muscles.

When glycogen is depleted through dietary restriction (or exercise), glucose synthesis or "gluconeogenesis" occurs by breaking down protein and other nutrients. Thus, adequate carbohydrate intake is essential in limiting the use of body protein (muscle) as an energy source.

FAT

Fats are compounds that contain carbon, hydrogen, and oxygen. Each gram of fat provides about 9 kcal. Fats are particularly dense in calories. For example, each of the following contains .1 kcal or 100 calories, the last three being "fatty" items: twenty stalks of celery, one medium potato, two cups of fresh strawberries, six ounces of white wine, one apple, eight large potato chips, one tablespoon butter or margarine, and two and a half teaspoons oil.

Triglyceride (glycerol and fatty acids cojoined) is the most abundant fat in the body. A fatty acid is said to be saturated when the carbons are "saturated" with hydrogens (i.e., the carbon atoms hold as many hydrogen atoms as possible). Some foods that contain saturated fatty acids are butter, red meats, coconut oil, and palm oil. Saturated fats tend to raise blood cholesterol levels. Unsaturated fatty acids liquify easily and tend to be liquids at room temperature. Examples of monounsaturated fatty acids are olive and peanut oils. Examples of polyunsaturated fatty acids (two or more double bonds along the main carbon chain) are corn and safflower oils.

Other groups of fat include phospholipids, important in blood clotting; cholesterol, present in all animal cells and important in the production of bile and reproductive hormones; and lipoproteins, responsible for transporting fat in the blood. Examples of lipoproteins include the high-density lipoproteins. These contain a relatively larger amount of protein and less cholesterol than their lower-density or LDL counterparts, and are responsible for returning cholesterol to the liver for disposal.

Fat represents a more compact or concentrated form of stored energy than glycogen. When glucose is stored as glycogen, 2.7 grams of water are required for each gram of glycogen on a dry-weight basis. This is one reason that there is an upper limit to the amount of glycogen that can be stored when athletes "glycogen load." Other important roles for fat are protection of vital organs and insulation of the body against external thermal stress.

PROTEIN

Protein contains carbon, hydrogen, and oxygen as well as nitrogen. It supplies energy, but has other roles: building blood, scar tissue, enzymes, hormones, and antibodies, and maintaining fluid and salt balance. Each gram of protein provides about 4 kcal. Proteins consist of amino acids, eight of which are considered essential (Essential Amino Acids or EAAs) because they must be obtained through the diet.

All foods contain protein because it is an important constituent of animal and plant cells, either structurally—to hold the cell together—or as enzymes which increase the rate of chemical reaction in the cell. Foods that contain relatively large amounts of water, such as vegetables and fruits, have small amounts of protein compared with breads, cereals, nuts, dried beans, and animal products.

A brain cell is only about 10 percent protein; muscle cells may contain over double that amount. Although resistance exercise encourages an increase in muscle size and protein content in exercised muscle, simply eating larger amounts of protein does not. In order for muscle cells to increase in size, a demand must be put on them (i.e., they must be made to work). Protein can't be "pushed" ("force-fed" with amino-acid supplements) into the cells, it must be "pulled" in—unlike fat, which is easily stored in the body when consumed in excess. Thus, there is no advantage to eating excess protein and doing so *may* ultimately be stressful on the liver and kidneys.

The RDA for protein is sufficiently high to cover most athletes' needs, but not unlike most Americans many athletes and dancers consume too much protein.[6] What athletes and dancers must ensure is sufficient *calorie* intake: to eat enough protein-sparing calories—carbohydrates—so that protein is not mobilized as an energy source.

Dancers take amino acids (e.g., protein powders) as supplements to meet dietary deficiencies and as ergogenic aids to build muscle, aid fat loss, and provide energy. However, there is little or no evidence that amino acid supplements will help them achieve these goals. In fact, "potential problems with excessive protein or amino acid intakes include excessive weight gain, dehydration, gout, and excessive loss of urinary calcium."[7] The supplements are also expensive.

The proteins contained in food are classified as complete or incomplete, depending on their amino acid composition. An incomplete, or lower-quality, protein is deficient in one or more of the EAAs. Foods predominant in the nonessential amino acids (NEAAs) should be consumed in larger amounts or complemented by foods high in the EAAs. For example, in wheat-based diets, the wheat must be consumed in portions larger than that which the American population would consider "normal" or consumed in combination with foods high in EAAs (e.g., low-fat dairy products). It makes sense, of course, that plant foods such as grains contain less of the EAAs than animal foods. For example, other animals share similar oxygen-transport systems; thus, humans have to eat fewer animal products to accumulate the requisite amino acids for the production of hemoglobin. This is not to say that the amino acids needed to produce hemoglobin cannot be derived from consumption of plants; it is just necessary to eat more and a greater variety of the plants.

It is easy to make complete proteins by combining different food groups.[8] From the *Legume Group*—beans (black, fava, kidney, lima, pinto, and so on), peas (black-eyed, chick, split), peanuts, and lentils; the *Grain Group*—barley, corn, oats, rice, wheat (wheat-germ, sprouts), flours, and cereals made from these grains; and the *Nut and Seed Group*—almonds, cashews, walnuts, pumpkin seeds, sesame seeds, sunflower seeds, and so on, the following combinations make complete proteins:

- Legumes and grains: rice-bean casserole, corn tortilla and beans, peanut butter sandwich
- Legumes and nuts or seeds: blended dips with garbanzo beans, lentil casserole
- Legumes and low-fat dairy products: cheese sauce for bean dish, enchiladas
- Grains and low-fat dairy products: cheese sandwich, sandwich with milk, rice pudding, pasta with cheese, pizza
- Nuts or seeds and low-fat dairy products: cottage cheese-nut croquettes
- Small amounts of meat, poultry, or fish and plant proteins

  These foods should be eaten preferably in their whole-grain, low-sodium, low-fat, or nonfat form.

When are our eating habits wasteful (i.e., amino acids are not used to build protein)? Amino acids are wasted when they are consumed in excess of the RDA, usually in high-fat, high-protein foods. Since protein cannot be stored as such, it is readily broken down and metabolized/stored for energy. However, an excess of anything is bound to get anyone in trouble, whether it is "red-meat" alternatives such as chicken or even the dancer's staple, carbohydrates (if eaten in large enough quantities, substantial amounts of protein and sodium can be consumed). What does one conclude from this? Everything in moderation; with perhaps one exception—water.

WATER

Water is hardly an energy nutrient, but it is essential for thermoregulation and for weight management. Very few dancers manage to consume the recommended sixty-four fluid ounces of water daily. The National Research Council recommends one milliliter (ml) per kcal of energy as an RDA for adults. According to the NRC, "The normal rate of turnover of water per day approximates six percent of total body weight in the adult. . . . The body is equipped with a number of homeostatic mechanisms . . . that operate to maintain total body water within narrow limits."[9] For an adult requiring about 2,000 kcal/day, the water consumption should be about 2,000 ml (2 liters).

For adequate hydration, at least twenty ounces of fluid should be consumed one or two hours before exercise, another ten to fifteen ounces fifteen minutes before exercise, and three to six ounces every ten to twenty minutes during exercise, regardless of whether or not one feels thirsty. Dehydration occurs long before thirst is experienced.

Because it is not possible for humans to adapt to inadequate water intake or excessive daily losses incurred through urine, feces, sweating, vomiting, dieting, diffusion through the skin, and exhalation of water vapor, dehydration inevitably results. Dehydration compromises the body's ability to function in many ways: by reducing muscular strength, lowering plasma and blood volumes, depleting liver glycogen stores, and so on. Basically, as a person sweats, body fluids are lost, which results in a lowered available volume of blood to provide oxygen and nutrients to working muscles and to deliver heat to the skin for body thermoregulation. As dehydration increases, the heart rate increases, the blood flow to the skin decreases, the body temperature increases, performance declines, and movement becomes labored. Even before pronounced thirst is experienced, the person may suffer fatigue, loss of coordination, irritability, and, in the very susceptible, cramps.

One adaptation to dehydration is sodium retention (the sweat becomes more diluted) as kidney production of the hormone aldosterone is increased. Repeated bouts of dehydration may cause the body to become more efficient at storing water in excess of the sweat loss, resulting in greater rehydration and "water-weight gain."[10]

Energy Expenditure: A Primer

Energy expenditure is a function of three factors: basal (BMR) or resting (RMR) metabolic rate; muscular activity; and assimilation of food, referred to as specific dynamic action/effect, dietary-induced thermogenesis, or thermic effect of feeding.

BMR is defined as the minimum level of energy needed to sustain the body's vital functions in the waking state. Technically, the BMR is usually determined by measuring oxygen consumption in a thermoneutral environment under very strict protocols. When the effects of temperature are not controlled in calorimetry studies (e.g., the subject is exercising at whatever the ambient room temperature is for that particular day), it is the RMR that is measured. The BMR is frequently misused to denote RMR in discussion of human thermoregulation. The RMR together with the thermic effect of feeding constitute what is called "resting energy metabolism."[11]

Muscular activity is the most variable component of energy expenditure and can constitute 15 to 30 percent of the daily total due to physical work, involuntary activity such as shivering and fidgeting, and purposeful physical exercise. Assimilation of food usually accounts for less than 10 percent of total calorie expenditure. Each type of energy nutrient—carbohydrate, fat, protein—has a different thermic effect. For example, the digestion of protein increases the metabolic rate dramatically because the liver expends quite a lot of energy processing the large amino acids.

Of the three factors, it is the RMR that represents the largest use of internal energy resources, accounting for about 70 percent of daily caloric expenditure. The beating of the heart, inhalation and exhalation of air, maintaining body temperature—these energy needs must be met before any calories are used for the other two factors.

There are many factors that influence RMR.[12] These include age (the younger the person, the higher the RMR); height (the taller the person, the larger the surface area, the more heat is lost from the surface of the skin, and thus the higher the RMR for maintaining body temperature); gender (males have higher RMRs than females owing to the presence of male sex hormones and to the higher percentage of lean body mass; muscle tissue is highly active, even at rest); health (fever increases the RMR of cells); fasting and/or constant malnutrition (RMR is lowered owing to loss of lean body tissue and the degeneration of body organs); and glandular secretions (such as the increase in RMR when epinephrine is released in response to stress).

Estimates of RMR can be made by using a nomogram.[13] The nomogram provides a simplified method for computing surface area based on height and weight. For example, I am about 5'6" and weigh 125 pounds. To determine my surface area, I would use the three scales of the nomogram to approximate 1.64 square meters. I would multiply 1.64 × 35 (38 for males) kcal/sq m/hr × 24 hrs to determine my daily RMR. Thus, I expend about 1,378 kcal daily just to sustain vital functions.

The RMR of a typical female dancer might be 1,100 kcal. If the dancer's caloric intake is low and basal metabolic needs are not being met, what adaptations does the body make? Besides becoming less active, which is usually not an option for dancers, one obvious change is that RMR decreases (i.e., the metabolism "slows down") and thus the need for calories declines. This is in large part due to the mobilization of lean body tissue as a source of energy. The only way to reverse the effect of severe caloric restriction, or depression of metabolic rate, is through exercise.[14]

Recommended Dietary Allowances (RDA)

RDA are defined as "The levels of intake of essential nutrients considered, in the judgment of the Committee on Dietary Allowances of the Food and Nutrition Board on the basis of available scientific knowledge, to be adequate to meet the known nutritional needs of practically all healthy persons."[15] The Committee emphasizes that these are not required amounts for any specific individual. Rather, they are *guidelines* for *healthy populations;* individuals with infections will experience increased metabolic losses of nitrogen and some vitamins and minerals and thus nutrient requirements will be higher.

The estimates (see Tables 7 and 8) are based on a number of techniques, including collection of data on nutrient intake from the food supply of healthy people, review of epidemiological studies when clinical consequences of nutrient deficiencies are found to be correctable by dietary improvement, biochemical measures that assess the degree of tissue saturation or adequacy of molecular function in relation to nutrient intake, nutrient balance studies that

Table 7. Adult RDA for Vitamins[a]

Vitamin	Sources	RDA	Comments
Fat Soluble			
A	Liver, fortified milk and margarine, butter, egg yolk, leafy green and yellow vegetables, dried apricots, cantaloupe, peaches, broccoli	800–1,000 RE[b]	Regular ingestion two to three times the RDA is not recommended
D	Fortified milk, eggs, fatty fish, liver, exposure to sunlight (approximately 15 minutes per day)	5–10 mcg	Vitamin D can be toxic if 2 to 10 times the RDA is ingested
E	Vegetable oils, wheat germ and whole grains, nuts, soybeans	8–10 mg	Toxicity reported at over 10 times the RDA (but reports are inconsistent)
K	Leafy green vegetables, cabbage, cauliflower, tomatoes, wheat bran	45–80 mg	
Water Soluble			
C	Citrus fruits, tomatoes, strawberries, melons, potatoes, broccoli, green peppers, kiwis, leafy vegetables	50–60 mg	Vitamin C in excess of 1 g/day may have a pharmacologic effect not related to the normal function of the vitamin

[a]Material in the table is from AHA (American Heart Association), *Heart Cuisine* (Los Angeles, Cal.: AHA, undated); Robin Chmelar and Sally Fitt, *Dancing at Your Peak: Diet* (Princeton, N.J.: Princeton Book Co., Publishers, 1990); Ellen Coleman, "Nutrition and weight control," in *Aerobic Dance-Exercise Instructor Manual*, Chapter 3 (San Diego, Cal.: IDEA Foundation, 1987); and NRC (National Research Council), *Recommended Dietary Allowances* (Washington, D.C.: National Academy Press, 1989).
[b]Key: RE = Retinol Equivalents; mcg = micrograms; mg = milligrams.

Table 7. Adult RDA for Vitamins (Continued)

Vitamin	Sources	RDA	Comments
Water Soluble (Continued)			
Thiamin	Pork, organ meats, legumes, whole-grain and enriched cereals and breads, wheat germ, lean meats and poultry, eggs	1.0–1.5 mg	
Riboflavin	Organ meats, milk and dairy products, whole-grain and enriched cereals and breads, eggs, fish, leafy vegetables	1.2–1.8 mg	Possible increased requirement during oral contraceptive usage
Niacin	Fish, liver, meat, poultry, eggs, peanuts, grains, legumes, brewer's yeast	13–20 mg	
Pyridoxine	Meat, cereal bran and germ, egg yolk, legumes, dry active yeast, sunflower seeds, beef liver, walnuts, salmon, bananas	1.4–2.0 mg	*Routine* supplementation for oral contraceptive users is not justified
B-12	Liver, kidney, meat, fish, clams, oysters, eggs	2.0 mcg	Bacterial contamination of centralized food supply also supplies some B-12

measure nutritional status in relation to intake, and studies of subjects maintained on diets containing low or deficient levels of a nutrient, followed by correction of the deficit with measured amounts of that nutrient (such studies are undertaken only when the risks to the subjects are minimal).

Once the data from the estimates are compiled and the

Table 7. Adult RDA for Vitamins (Continued)

Vitamin	Sources	RDA	Comments
Water Soluble (Continued)			
Folacin	Green vegetables, organ meats, lean beef, eggs, fish, dry beans, lentils, asparagus, wheat germ and bran, brewer's yeast, orange juice, almonds, bananas	150–200 mcg	
Pantothenic Acid	Whole-grain cereals, organ meats, eggs, vegetables, liverwurst, chicken, tomato sauce, sweet potatoes, white potatoes	4–7 mg	
Biotin	Liver, egg yolk, peanuts, yeast, milk, legumes, bananas, cereal, mushrooms, meat, most vegetables, grapefruit, tomato, watermelon, strawberries	30–100 mcg	

recommended level of nutrient intake is indicated, the requirement is increased by an amount sufficient to meet the needs of all members of the population and to take into account inefficient utilization by the body of the nutrient (e.g., iron). The RDA, by necessity, then represent rather generous recommendations because estimated average requirements are increased to take into account individual biological variability.

Given the methods used to determine the RDA and the

Table 8. Adult RDA for Minerals and Trace Elements[a]

Mineral	Sources	RDA
Calcium	Milk and milk products, dark green leafy vegetables, broccoli, sardines, clams, oysters	800–1,200 mg[b]
Phosphorus	Meat, fish, poultry, legumes, milk and milk products, whole-grain cereals	800–1,200 mg
Magnesium	Whole grains, nuts, dark leafy vegetables, grains, legumes, meat, milk	270–400 mg

Trace Element[c]	Sources	RDA
Iron	Liver, red meat, fish, poultry, legumes, whole grains, dried fruit, dark green leafy vegetables, blackstrap molasses, potatoes	10–15mg
Zinc	Liver, shellfish, eggs, meat, milk, herring, wheat bran	12–15 mg
Iodine	Iodized table salt, seafood, water, dairy products	150 mcg
Copper	Liver, kidney, shellfish, oysters, whole grains, nuts, legumes, chocolate	1.5–3.0 mg
Manganese	Nuts and unrefined grains, vegetables, fruits	2.5–5.0 mg
Fluoride	Fluoridated water, coffee, tea, soybeans, spinach, gelatin, onion, lettuce	1.5–4.0 mg

[a]Material in the table is from AHA (American Heart Association), *Heart Cuisine* (Los Angeles, Cal.: AHA, undated); Robin Chmelar and Sally Fitt, *Dancing at Your Peak: Diet* (Princeton, N.J.: Princeton Book Co., Publishers, 1990); Ellen Coleman, "Nutrition and weight control," in *Aerobic Dance-Exercise Instructor Manual,* Chapter 3 (San Diego, Cal.: IDEA Foundation, 1987); and NRC (National Research Council), *Recommended Dietary Allowances* (Washington, D.C.: National Academy Press, 1989).
[b]Key: mg = milligrams; mcg = micrograms.
[c]For the first time, the RDA (40 to 70 mcg) has been set for selenium, a trace element that functions as part of an enzyme. The enzyme acts as an antioxidant.

assumptions that must be made in that determination, it is not surprising that the allowances are not considered permanent. They are revised at approximately five-year intervals, as additional data are made available. The 1989 RDA, published four years later than the projected release date, reflect significant changes from the 1980 RDA: the calcium level is increased from 800 mg/day to 1,200 mg for men and women age nineteen to twenty-four (previously, the 1,200 mg recommendation applied only to eleven- to eighteen-year-olds); the RDA for vitamin C is increased for adults who smoke; 500 mg/day of sodium is established as a "safe minimum"; and for the first time the RDA for vitamin K and selenium have been set.

An underlying assumption of the determinations is that food selections will be made from a wide variety of choices. This is to ensure that nutrients that are known to be required, but for which no RDA have been established, are consumed in sufficient quantities.

Under no circumstances should the RDA be used as justification for reducing habitual intakes of nutrients. Likewise, they are not meant to be met with extensive vitamin and mineral supplementation or by megafortification of single foods. When vitamins and minerals are indicated for supplementation, they are meant to supplement a somewhat robust daily diet: that does not mean a carton of yogurt, half a sandwich, a salad, and an apple.

The body will adapt to occasional periods of nutrient deprivation. This is why, in estimating dietary adequacy, it is acceptable to average intakes over a five- to eight-day period. However, food supplementation on a regular basis is not recommended. One of the main reasons for this is that macronutrients (protein, carbohydrates) cannot be supplemented. Carbohydrates are required in large amounts (accounting for at least 50 percent of total calories), as is protein (approximately forty to sixty grams per day, or 12 to 15 percent of total calories).

As some food scientists note:

> While significant progress has been achieved in developing technological approaches to particular micronutrient deficiencies . . . the attempt to devise technological solutions to macronutrient deficiencies such as protein entails problems of a completely different magnitude. . . . macronutrient deficits (whether protein or protein-calorie) require consumption in relatively large, daily quantities. As a result, the medical-type intervention [supplements as "medication"] as a response to

macrodeficits is rendered totally inappropriate. Protein or protein-calorie interventions can only be conceived to be what they actually are, [i.e.] sources of food, with all of the social, cultural, and economic preferences and constraints that this involves.[16]

Supplements cannot be treated as medicines, as drugs, as a shot of this, or a hit of that. Dancers must adopt a new paradigm of eating, not "I need some vitamin A or thiamine or protein," but "I need to eat enough carbohydrates to meet my calorie and other nutrient needs." Adequate carbohydrate intake—assuming a wide variety of complex carbohydrates—ensures adequate intake of various nutrients (see Tables 7 and 8) and of protein.[17]

Energy intake must be of primary concern, as suggested by the National Research Council (NRC): "It is . . . difficult to assure nutritional adequacy of diets that are low in energy content (less than 1,800–2,000 kcal) unless fats, sugar, and alcohol are more rigidly restricted than is customary in most American households."[18]

Recommended Intakes of Energy Nutrients

Carbohydrates should constitute at least 55 to 65 percent of daily caloric intake. A diet devoid of carbohydrates is likely to lead to ketosis (see Glossaries). This can be prevented by consuming about 50 to 100 grams of carbohydrate every day. However, intakes above this minimal level are recommended.

The NRC notes that intake of complex carbohydrates should be increased to replace the calories lost by reducing fat consumption. The Council recommends consumption of five or more servings (half-cup = one serving) every day of vegetables and fruits, especially green and yellow vegetables and citrus fruits, and at least six daily servings of grains and legumes.

Potatoes, grains, and beans (without cheese and/or sour cream) compared with meats are not high-calorie foods. The following are given by the American Heart Association (AHA)[19]:

Food	Calories
Boiled potato, one medium	106
White rice, one cup	153
Kidney beans, 3/4 cup	165
Spaghetti, one cup	210

Dietary fiber is the residue of plant food resistant to human digestive enzymes. No RDA have been set for fiber, although one will see guidelines of six grams of crude fiber or fifteen to thirty grams of dietary fiber. This is easy to obtain by eating two-thirds cup of cornflakes or shredded wheat biscuits for breakfast, a sandwich for lunch, an apple and a peach for "snacks," and baked beans or corn on the cob for dinner as part of the daily food intake.

No more than 30 percent of caloric intake should be in the form of *fat* (10 percent polyunsaturated, 10 percent monounsaturated, and no more than 10 percent saturated). A diet containing fifteen to twenty-five grams of food fats will usually meet the dietary requirement for fat-soluble vitamins and essential fatty acids (primarily linoleic).

Note that dietary fat is present in "visible fats," such as butter, lard, mayonnaise, cooking oil, and external fat on meats, as well as in "invisible fats," such as milk, cheese, meats, cereals, and breads (even bread contains one to two grams of fat per slice, but when the slice of bread has one-half tablespoon of butter on it the food jumps to almost seven grams of fat). For example, the percentage of total calories from fat is given by the AHA[20]:

Crackers	40	Hot dog (no roll)	80
Italian dressing	98	Cheese (cheddar)	72
Walnuts (shelled)	85	French fries	43

The AHA adds recommendations to reduce fat content:

- Choose lean meat, fish, and poultry. (Even though the beef is lean, three ounces of cooked, untrimmed, boneless sirloin compared with one and a half cups of cooked legumes such as navy beans contains 27.2 grams of fat compared with 1.5 grams for the legumes; the protein content—20 grams—and calories are the same.)
- Limit intake of saturated fats (butter, cream, hydrogenated fats in margarine and shortening).
- Broil, bake, poach, steam instead of fry.
- Use a minimum of fats and oils in cooking.
- Use moderate amounts of monounsaturated oils for flavoring.
- Read food labels carefully to determine the amount and type of fat contained in a product.

Protein should account for no more than 10 to 15 percent of total caloric intake.[21] Corrections in the calculation of the RDA are made to take into account the utilization of protein in a mixed diet. Thus, the RDA for the mixed animal and plant proteins typical of the United States diet are 0.8 g/kg of body weight per day. The allowance for a 70 kg (154 lb.) man would be fifty-six grams of protein per day; for a 56 kg (123 lb.) woman, forty-five grams.

There is little evidence that muscular activity increases the need for protein. Although coaches quite often recommend 1.0 gram or higher per kilogram of body weight for an athlete, the NRC adds no such increment for training. The reason for this is that *if* professional athletes need additional protein, it is in ample supply in the extra calories consumed in high-carbohydrate foods.

Diet and Weight Control

The Importance of Carbohydrates

For the general population—and dancers are no exception—most of the calories in the diet should come from carbohydrates because foods high in carbohydrates also contain ample amounts of vitamins and minerals. As long as dancers consume enough varied complex carbohydrates (and water), nutrient deficiences should be uncommon. This may be a tall order. Bonbright has reported that even though dancers consumed close to their RDA for calories (83.7 percent of the RDA), the RDA for biotin, zinc, linoleic acid, copper, iodine, and chloride were not met. Almost all the dancers were deficient in the other vitamins and minerals studied, with the exception of B-2, B-1, C, B-3, A, K, B-12, sodium, and chromium.[22]

The body needs carbohydrates to provide a continuous supply of energy to the cells. The carbohydrates in food eventually break down in digestion into simple sugar units or glucose.

Glucose is one of the two major fuels used by the cells for energy (the other is fatty acids). Glucose is usually the only fuel source for the brain and central nervous system. Glucose levels in the blood are maintained by periodic eating of foods containing carbohydrates and by release of glucose from stored glycogen. A small percentage of glucose can be obtained from amino acids (the "building blocks" of protein) in muscles and other tissue proteins—this percentage dramatically increases during carbohydrate deprivation.

The brain alone requires about 400 to 600 kcal each day as glucose. Even at rest, it consumes about two-thirds of the total circulating blood glucose. What happens when dancers deprive their bodies of calories, especially of carbohydrates?

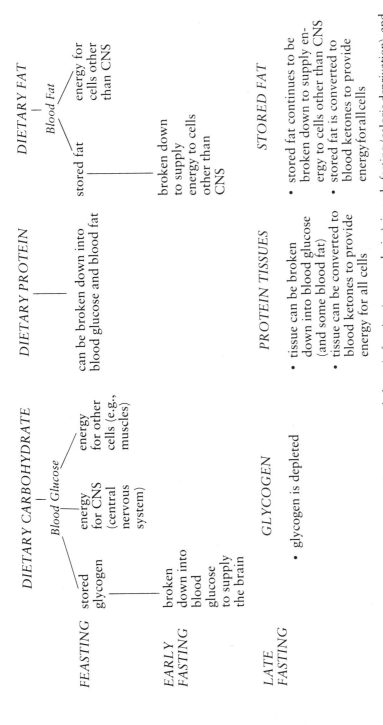

Figure 38. Energy flow in feasting and fasting: energy balance in feasting (excess calories), in early fasting (calorie deprivation), and in late fasting (severe caloric deprivation). (*Adapted from E. M. Hamilton, E. N. Whitney, and F. S. Sizer, Nutrition: Concepts and Controversies. 3rd ed. [St. Paul, Minn.: West Publishing Co., 1985]*)

DIETARY CARBOHYDRATE

Blood Glucose

energy for CNS (central nervous system)

energy for other cells (e.g., muscles)

FEASTING   stored glycogen

EARLY FASTING   broken down into blood glucose to supply the brain

LATE FASTING

GLYCOGEN

• glycogen is depleted

DIETARY PROTEIN

can be broken down into blood glucose and blood fat

PROTEIN TISSUES

• tissue can be broken down into blood glucose (and some blood fat)
• tissue can be converted to blood ketones to provide energy for all cells

---

DIETARY FAT

Blood Fat

energy for cells other than CNS

stored fat

broken down to supply energy to cells other than CNS

STORED FAT

• stored fat continues to be broken down to supply energy to cells other than CNS
• stored fat is converted to blood ketones to provide energy for all cells

Feasting and Fasting

In the first few days of a fast, tissue protein provides most of the needed energy, the remainder coming from fat reserves (see Fig. 38, "late fasting"). The loss of protein can usually be controlled by exercise and carbohydrate consumption.[23]

Without adequate carbohydrate intake, death would inevitably result were it not for a specific metabolic adaptation: ketosis. In ketosis, the body converts fatty acid (fat) and amino acid (protein) fragments into ketone bodies, a fuel alternative to glucose, thus allowing the body to survive an extended period of starvation or "self-induced" starvation. If ketone bodies are produced in excess of what can be excreted in the urine, however, they can accumulate in the blood, leading to "acidosis."

The adult body thus adapts to a carbohydrate deprivation/ starvation situation by mobilizing amino acids (which decreases muscle mass), degrading the organs (in particular, the liver), and decreasing resting or basal metabolism. This is obviously helpful for people who are trying to survive a famine situation; it is exceptionally counterproductive to dancers who want to "lose weight" quickly and permanently. The body begins to *need* fewer calories because fat tissue requires considerably fewer to maintain itself than does muscle. Moreover, because certain organs begin to waste away, the body is not capable of performing as much work and therefore requires fewer calories for daily maintenance.

How Do Diets "Work"?

Low-calorie, low-carbohydrate diets work in terms of *short-term* weight loss. In fact, some hospitals administer VLC diets (very low calorie, 400–800 kcal/day: a "modified fast") in which the patients are strictly monitored; five-pound losses per week are common. These diets do not work in terms of *long-term* weight management. Most of the weight that is lost on the bathroom scale is from mobilizing protein and water. Approximately 75 percent of the weight lost during the first week of the diet is water, the rest coming mostly from muscle tissue.[24]

With a low-carbohydrate intake, the body must use its meagre stores of glycogen for fuel. Water is needed to store glycogen; when glycogen is depleted, so is the water stored with it. Muscle itself is about 70 percent water, which further explains the obligatory water loss that accompanies muscle breakdown.

When refeeding starts, the body restores its glycogen stores and fat deposits first, so that the first weight regained is water (for the storage of glycogen) and fat. This is why starvation dieters regain weight with a greater proportion of the regained weight as fat.

Another risk is that, with repeated or "yo-yo" dieting, the fat or adipose cells adapt by becoming increasingly efficient at storing fatty acids. Thus, it is even harder to lose weight during the next dieting bout or to retain the loss of those 7 or 10 pounds for any extended time period. Of course, dancers with rigorous work schedules have an activity level sufficiently high to force the body to use fat as an energy reserve, but their slim, lithe body may belie a large percentage of internal fat, possibly as an adaptation to repeated dieting bouts. Nevertheless, dancers continue to "yo-yo" diet. In one study, Bonbright found that 37.5 percent of the dancers interviewed dieted five or more times a year for twelve-day periods.[25]

Fortunately, our body is "smart." We are relieved of calculating percentages and weights for the appropriate amount of protein, fat, and carbohydrates in our diet—to some extent. Excess calories as protein, fat, or simple carbohydrates are readily converted to fats. But as complex carbohydrates they are less likely to be converted for a variety of reasons, principally that it is difficult to eat complex carbohydrates in excess and that the energy cost of storing them as fat is greater than, for example, of storing fat as fat. Alternatively, if the diet is deficient in carbohydrates, protein and fat will eventually be converted to ketone bodies.

Fat Management

It is easy to become fixated on day-to-day "weight" fluctuations on the scale. However, dancers' primary concern should be their body *composition*—their relative amounts of fat and muscle. It is well known that dance is a "low body fat" profession, with female professional dancers ranging from 11 to 16 percent body fat and male professional dancers ranging from 5 to 11 percent.[26] These figures are low, compared with values averaging over 12 percent for men and 20 percent for women in the general population.

How is it possible to reduce the percentage of fat in the body? How can fat be mobilized as an energy source? It is thought that the best way is through low-intensity exercise. This "light" exercise applies just the right amount of stress to energy systems so that the slow lipolysis ("fat-splitting") process can take place.

During exercise intensities demanding more than 50 to 60

percent of the maximal oxygen uptake, muscle glycogen is the major fuel—its depletion coincides with the time of exhaustion. However, as the duration of the exercise increases to several hours, more than 50 percent of the energy is supplied by fat. Blood glucose also increases in importance as an energy source during prolonged exercise.[27]

For example, a mail carrier will have used by the end of the day 90 percent of his or her energy as fat. Just sitting in a chair or sleeping—both considered "light" activity—will cause a large percentage of the fuel to be mobilized as fat.

The *total* amount of fuel used in "light" activity, however, will be low compared with the amount used in intense activity, such as repeated jumping. For the jumping activity ("moderate" to "heavy" exercise), energy requirements are higher. Although a smaller percentage of the fuel will be derived from fat *during the exercise,* especially if it is of short duration (glycogen and circulating blood glucose are used first), total fat mobilized postexercise may be substantial and the physiological effects of such exercise may be long-lasting.

There are at least three reasons for this: (1) Up to eight hours after exercise, the body's metabolic rate, and thus need for calories, remains elevated. (2) Because exercise that sufficiently stresses the body's musculoskeletal system may result in muscle accretion and thus an increase in lean body mass, the body's metabolic rate remains slightly elevated, assuming that the exercise is rigorous. More energy is required to maintain a gram of muscle than a gram of fat, but also more energy is required to *build* the protein. Synthesis of protein is energetically expensive. Several hours after exercise, protein synthesis increases and remains elevated up to twenty-four hours.[28] (3) Glucose tolerance is increased for several days after vigorous exercise, partly owing to the increased glucose uptake by muscle in order to replenish glycogen stores.

One does not have to look very far for tables that illustrate how many kcal one can "burn" during a specific exercise. For example, for a 123-pound person, the following energy expenditure can be expected:[29]

Archery	216 kcal per hour
Badminton	324 kcal per hour
Swimming, backstroke	570 kcal per hour
Dance technique class	200–300 kcal per hour

Such charts are virtually useless unless one separates the data for gender, weight, and so on. Worse, they feed our society's obsession with the "quick fix": "I ate a brownie, so now I'll get on an exercise bike for forty-five minutes to work it off."

Physiologically, the only given in terms of "burning" energy is that phosphorus-containing energy compounds (called adenosine triphosphate, or ATP) must be broken down to release energy. If one wants to manipulate the fuels (fat, carbohydrate) from which the compounds are formulated, the body must be conditioned in terms of number and size of mitochondria (the cell's "powerhouse" unit), oxidative enzymes, and muscle fiber type.[30]

In addition, the duration of and nutritional intake before exercising determine which fuel source will be most easily mobilized. For example, consuming glucose less than an hour before exercising encourages the body to use glucose rather than fat as a fuel source, all other factors being equal. Again, biophysical and chemical inertia take over in determining how much fat is "burned."

The bottom line is that if calories are going to be somewhat restricted (not to fall below 1,500 kcal daily, mostly in the form of carbohydrates), the individual has to engage in daily endurance activity for at least thirty minutes to restrict muscle loss. Thus, only through balanced food intake and daily endurance activity will the effects of severe caloric deprivation—the metabolic changes that result from the loss of muscle and organ tissue—be reversed.

DIETING: AN OBSESSION

Most dancers are obsessed with dieting. There is a diet mentality that is pervasive in dance and in our society at large: food becomes an obsession. People eat virtually nothing all day only to eat with abandon in the evening.[31] Once a "forbidden food" is eaten and the dieter has "failed," even more "forbidden foods" are eaten. Stringent practice quotas may be self-imposed, specifying how many calories are to be expended each day.

Dancers have to develop a more realistic attitude toward food. Of course, it is frightening to relinquish faith in "controls": wearing tight clothes, daily weighings-in, or labeling foods as "good" and "bad." The way to gain control of the obsession, however, is to relinquish the notion of diet—calorie restriction—and return to normal eating habits, trying to follow the guidelines given above and letting the body's physiological hunger cues govern what and how much is eaten. Weight goals must be realistic.

Carbohydrate Management

SPACING MEALS

The spacing and scheduling of meals is a problem for dancers. As ABT's Cynthia Harvey says, "Most of the time, I really don't eat three meals a day, although I know that when I do I'm better off. In fact, I went to a nutritionist who told me I'd be better off eating six tiny meals a day for my metabolism."[32] This advice is well taken. The three-meal daily diet is a result of cultural conditioning, not physiological necessity.

Dancers are busy, constantly working. They take class, rehearse, perform, teach class, tour. As one dancer said, "When I tour, my diet is anything but sublime." In colleges and universities, students go to class, choreograph, rehearse, perform, take notes, sit for exams, write papers, dance more, study. It's hard to find time to eat.

In the battle for consumption of different food groups—simple carbohydrates, complex carbohydrates, fat, and protein—there is no contest. The winners are clearly simple carbohydrates (sugary foods), fats (fatty, baked foods), and protein-fats (meats and cheeses). With the exception of pasta, most complex carbohydrates in the form of breads, cereals, and potatoes play a minor role in the dancer's daily diet.

Generally, dancers don't eat regularly. They grab whatever they can, usually foods high in fat and salt. Dancer Peter Fonseca says:

> What I try to do is get used to functioning at a high energy level all day long with as little eating as possible. I mean, within reason of course, not trying to starve myself. If I can get to the point where I am used to smaller amounts of food, it gets easier.[33]

For most dancers, it is difficult to schedule full meals consisting of a varied diet. However, it doesn't matter: if at least 900 carbohydrate-rich kcal are not consumed on a daily basis,[34] the body will compensate by degrading dietary protein and muscle tissue for the needed glucose—no matter what the dancer puts into or purges from the body.

TIMING IS EVERYTHING

Eating most of the daily calories at one time rather than spacing meals throughout the day can result in large swings in blood glucose levels, intense hunger contractions, and overconsumption of foods high in sugar and fat. The blood glucose level is regulated by a number of hormones, including insulin. Most carbohydrates are absorbed relatively quickly, producing a sudden increase in blood glucose. When this happens, glucose is easily diffused into cells. As insulin is released, the liver and other cells are stimulated to convert glucose to glycogen and fat, and the breakdown of fats and proteins is temporarily inhibited.

After long periods—up to six hours—without food, blood glucose levels drop dramatically. Nerve cells in the brain (hypothalamus) detect this condition of deprivation and generate nerve impulses that signal hunger to the conscious part of the brain: the cortex. (The headache that might occur can be alleviated by eating sugar.[35]) Stomach contractions intensify concurrent with a craving for carbohydrates.

It is thus better to eat a full sandwich for lunch than try to do without food altogether. What dancers should not do, but usually do, is eat practically nothing—a little salad, a half bagel, some yogurt—generally thinking of food all day long but resisting eating until hunger is so great that they will eat anything in sight. This usually means eating something high in sugar or fat for rapid satiety. Actually, in a hunger-panic situation, given a choice of a high-fat or high-sugar food, eating sugar is a better nutritional choice.

There is no argument that it is best to spread sugar loads throughout the day to avoid becoming hyperglycemic or hypoglycemic. However much sugar is maligned,[36] if dancers do not suffer from dental caries or diabetes and do consume adequate dietary fiber, vitamins, and minerals, sugary foods are preferred over fat. Good luck, though, finding sugary foods that are not loaded with fat, other than soft drinks and some candies. Still, if necessary, it's better to eat a hard candy (floss teeth afterward!) than a Haägen-Dazs ice cream bar.

When the body is deprived of food, it seems to call upon every psychological and physiological mechanism at its disposal to drive itself to eat. A one-meal-a-day schedule will certainly increase appetite. Dancers pass up food they really want in order to keep their weight down, and then "pig out," eating beyond satiety. This is part of the obsession with food, insulin levels notwithstanding. Instead, what dancers should focus on is how to distribute their caloric intake throughout the day with complex carbohydrates. To this end, there are certain foods that dancers should incorporate into their diet that are high in calories from carbohydrates, yet low in sodium and saturated fat (Table 9).

Table 9. Foods High in Calories from Carbohydrates and Relatively Low in Saturated Fats*

Hot Cereal: cereal cooked with water or nonfat (preferable to low-fat) milk. Add small amounts of peanut butter, sunflower seeds, wheat germ, or dried fruit.

Toast: spread lightly with jelly or jam, low-sodium margarine, or peanut butter (nuts and nut butters should be consumed in moderation).

Salads: low-calorie salads are converted into full meals by adding low-sodium, low-fat cottage cheese, garbanzo beans, sunflower seeds, vegetables, chopped walnuts, tuna fish (high-protein foods such as tuna fish should be consumed in moderation), low-sodium croutons.

Soups (all low-sodium): hearty lentil, split pea, minestrone, and barley.

Sandwiches: hearty, dense breads (such as thick-sliced sprouted wheat), stuffed with tuna salad, bean spreads, or lightly spread with nut butters.

Desserts: low-sodium oatmeal raisin cookies, rice pudding, fruit compotes, low-sodium muffins, and sweet breads.

Snacks: fruit yogurts, bananas, sandwiches.

*Nancy Clark, "How to increase calorie intake," *The Physician and Sportsmedicine* 16/6 (1988): 140. The foods in this table do not comprise a daily diet; rather, they should *supplement* a daily diet already rich in complex carbohydrates.

— *Profiles* —

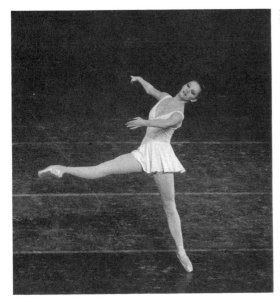

Photo courtesy © Steven Caras, 1990

Judith Fugate

Judith Fugate sees a lot of dancers at NYCB who are working "beyond their limits." True, the technique required to dance Balanchine's ballets is very fast-paced. The dancers must have the strength before they can find the speed. For Fugate, this has been an especially slow process, but it has paid off.

In 1986, at age twenty-nine, Fugate was promoted to principal status. She had started dancing at the age of two, and began her studies at SAB at age nine. At seventeen, she was taken into the company, and at twenty-four was promoted to soloist. Fugate made slow but steady progress. She has seen many dancers come and go. Even today, she is "amazed at the number of people in the company who do not work well." Out of 120 people she sees in her classes, only a handful are careful about how they work.

Fugate feels that it is important to have some ideas about principles of kinesiology, proper technique, and alignment before the dancer takes a daily company class. She has specific suggestions:

- Although demi-pliés are not a problem, one should avoid

grands pliés, especially in any position other than second; otherwise, too much stress is put on the knees.
- Fondu is the basis of most movements in ballet. This must be performed very clearly with the spine neutral as it moves up and down. You really have to be careful about hyperextending and losing the neutrality of the spine, it's so important.

She also talks about taking responsibility for one's own body. This extends to many different areas, not only technique but also diet, layoffs, and relaxation. She admits that anorexia is a problem in the company, similar to other ballet companies. She says, "Most dancers think about how much they are eating, not what. This is a problem, so many of the female dancers do not have a very feminine physique. They're so thin." There's no doubt that professional ballet is a difficult life:

> So many dancers are disillusioned. There are very few financial rewards in ballet. The work is so hard—class in the morning, rehearsal for five to six hours, then dancing in two to three ballets, six nights a week. Especially for the corps, it's very difficult, but the artistic rewards make all the hard work worth it. I know, I was there.
>
> Many dancers at SAB with me completely gave it up. There are only a certain number of positions in professional ballet companies, and even when you're at the top there are only a certain number of roles among the principals. There is a huge, big dance world out there beyond NYCB, but most of the dancers can't see beyond what's in the theatre. I feel those dancers who are not so "tunnel-visioned" are more successful with their careers.
>
> I guess what I'm saying is that even at NYCB, in the company, you still have to see all the possibilities, you have to look out for yourself, and especially, be very, very careful how you work. You have to watch that spine, and not sacrifice your alignment for a look or for an ideal. If you need to do that, then it's time for some extracurricular strengthening and stretching work.

• • • • • • • • • • • • • • • •

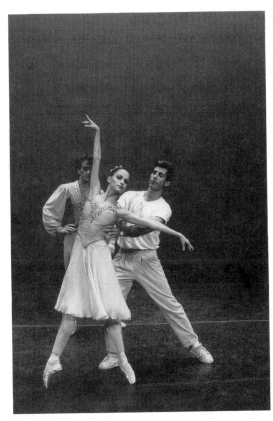

Photo courtesy © Leslie Sternlieb, 1990

Steven Caras

Many people know Steven Caras as an internationally acclaimed dance photographer. His photographs appear regularly in major publications, including the *New York Times, Newsweek, Time,* the *Los Angeles Times, Vogue, Dance Magazine,* and *Life.* Perhaps they've seen one of the seven books that feature his photographs, among which are *Peter Martins: Prince of the Dance, Balanchine: Photo Album and Memoir,* and *Ballet Life Behind the Scenes.* But there is also Steven Caras the dancer. Caras performed for fourteen years with NYCB.

Throughout his career, he has danced featured roles in many Balanchine and Robbins ballets, including the principal male dancer in *Agon, The Four Temperaments, The Nutcracker, The Dybbuk, Fanfare, The Goldberg Variations, Valse Fantaisie,* and *Donizetti Variations.* Jerome Robbins created one of the four principal male roles in *Scherzo Fantastique* on him for the ballet's premiere.

Caras has also coached dancers at all levels of training in

companies that include NYCB, Pennsylvania Ballet Company, and Ballet Oklahoma. As ballet master with Miami City Ballet, he is involved in the company's newly formed apprentice program as well as being Miami City Ballet's resident photographer.

What is his advice to professional dancers, to those who want a lifetime in dance? He reflects on his professional dance career:

> What I wish I had done when I was younger was to be more balanced in my diet. Instead, I'd go for hours without eating something, saving up for "the big reward—a big dinner." My mentality when I was young was that if I didn't eat, I'd be thin; if I ate five times a day, I'd get fat. But dancers should know that they can eat five times a day, maintaining a consistent weight they're comfortable with.
>
> Dancers should eat frequently throughout the day. Now that I'm thirty-nine, I'm in better shape than I was at eighteen or twenty-one. When I was younger, I didn't listen to older dancers and teachers—I thought I had it all mapped out for myself.

Caras also believes that dancers must condition their bodies in order to dance well: "I was dancing my very best when I was doing Pilates. More exercise 'around dancing' is essential. . . . I've done situps my whole life; I learned how to do them *correctly* just this year. The new kinds of crunches people are doing are the best. Teachers are just learning how to teach them."

While acknowledging that no two dancers are exactly alike in terms of their conditioning and nutritional needs, technical skills, rehearsal schedules, and performance repertory, he does suggest what a work day might look like for a dancer "nutritionally in balance," for example, for a member of the NYCB corps:

- Morning: If one has an appetite in the morning, it's wonderful to eat a lot. Breakfast might consist of a piece of fruit; coffee or tea—just a little caffeine; and oatmeal, maybe with honey, bananas, or sugar.
- Company class: An hour or so after breakfast, I was usually in company class. Some people warm up before the class and some people don't. In my warm-up, I start with stomach exercises. These are a good foundation for the warm-up and for the rest of the day—like a good breakfast. Stretching should be done only after the body is warm.
- Rehearsal: Company class was usually from 11:00 to 12:00. Right after that, there would be a two- to

three-hour rehearsal. After all this dancing, I found that I needed to eat something substantial—a sandwich and some fruit perhaps.

- Pre- and post-performance: When I wasn't on until the last ballet of the evening, a meal at 3:00 P.M. wouldn't have been enough to get me through the rest of the day and the performance. I would need to eat something again around 6:00 P.M. After the performance, I'd eat something very light—I couldn't go from 6:00 P.M. to 8:00 A.M. the next morning without eating anything.

What all this means is that to keep his energy level consistent throughout those long days, he'd have to eat smaller meals more frequently.

Six

Taking Control

Dancers usually have little control over powerful external forces in their lives: manipulative dance teachers, authoritative school directors, company/audience expectations.[1] Eating endless carbohydrates, lifting weights, and icing inflamed tendons will not make everything beautiful at the ballet. Far from it. As one specialist in the field told me:

> I must say, personally, that I am not quite as optimistic as you are; namely, I really don't feel that dancers have that much control over their own situation. It's one thing for a soloist or a principal dancer to call the shots, but corps dancers in professional companies just don't have those kinds of opportunities, and until the dance world accepts its responsibilities, young corps dancers as well as student dancers will always be victimized.

Clearly, in the business of dance, dancers are commodities—useful things to be bought and sold, bartered, and exchanged. They own few resources except their own labor, although some of them try to produce their own work. The reality is that it's a buyer's market, cutting across all idioms and production/employment situations: ballet, modern, jazz, theatre, show, nightclub, educational, or ethnic dance; professional and semiprofessional soloist or ensemble dancers and choreographers.

Some employment situations allow for much stronger dancer-control than others. Nevertheless, a lot of trying to "make it" in dance is going to be a struggle: to get into a company, to stay, to get challenging roles, to have a decent salary and working conditions, to find good teaching jobs, to produce dance, to create and actualize an aesthetic that may be counter to what is commercially viable or palatable to the general public. Dancers must find a balance in their lives among self-respect, self-fulfillment, and a reasonable salary.

In order to do this, they must clarify their values and goals. They must ask questions—the same questions that will be asked and discussed throughout this chapter:

- Why dance (how strong is the desire)?
- Who should dance (are there limitations)?
- How to dance (where to train, what are appropriate body image/metaphors for dance education)?
- What to dance (whose choreography)?
- What to earn and under what working conditions?

Power and longevity come from knowledge about health, nutrition, strength training, and conditioning, but dancers also need information on collective bargaining, relative salaries in the dance world, and work conditions in dance and other performing arts.

Once the questions are asked and answered, it's time for dancers to take assertive action. This may mean negotiating contracts (with union support), soliciting local public sympathies for more funds, or perhaps writing a letter to the dean, president, and/or board of directors of a college when the department chair has capriciously dismissed dance faculty. Some possible courses of action are suggested in this chapter.

Why Dance?

Professional dancers must really want to dance to stay with it, since dance is so emotionally and physically demanding. The competition is fierce. There's not much work, and what there is is poorly paid. It's expensive to produce. For some, it's a question of inertia: they have spent so many years learning and maturing, why throw it all away? For others, dancing is their passion: they continue to dance as long as the joy and excitement of performing outweigh the physical demands of preparation.

Clearly, the push factors—poor pay and exhausting rehearsal and performing schedules—aren't as strong as possible pull factors—the fierce and unconditional passion and excitement for the work, the need for a creative outlet, the status and prestige, the challenging repertory. Few dancers experience all of these pull factors in their lifetime. They don't have to; the joy of performing overshadows the harsh realities of dance and allows them to dream of alternative realities and visions.

It is these alternatives that need to take form as dancers' rights—the right to respect, to financial remuneration (always a function of market forces in our economy), to creative and artistic license, to work in a safe environment. Dancers of all ages, shapes, sizes, and idioms must work hard in between hours of training and rehearsal to establish and maintain these rights.

Who Should Dance?

Dance is for everyone. A prime example of that principle in action is in Washington, D.C., where Liz Lerman's Dance Exchange works together with Dancers of the Third Age, whose company members range in age from sixty to ninety and come from diverse ethnic backgrounds (Fig. 39). Almost the only thing that these dancers have in common is their desire to dance professionally. They transcend stereotypes and fads, refusing to be pigeonholed or dismissed as aerobicizing seniors. Instead, they serve as role models for the physically and artistically active, challenging anyone who wishes to dance to do so—recreationally or professionally—and thus redefine for audiences what dance is and who dancers are.

Lerman tries to keep in touch with this desire to dance:

> I am interested in remembering why I started to dance and how happy I was at that moment; in what we dance about; in who gets to do the dancing . . . in keeping professional dancers alive as human beings. In [a] time when people . . . are too fat, too clumsy, too old, too sick to dance, [everyone must step out and dance. Both] the dancer and the watcher [are transformed] in that moment.[2]

Lerman is committed to the idea that performance dance is generous, that it can accommodate *all* dancers who want to work. It is not the exclusive domain of a youthful professional elite. Likewise, that same professional elite should not feel overwhelmed and

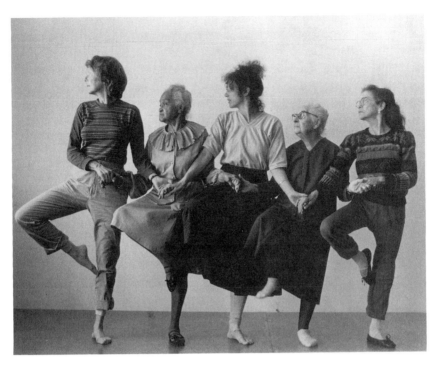

Figure 39. Liz Lerman *(center)* performing with Dancers of the Third Age. *(Photo by Dennis Deloria. Photo © The Dance Exchange, 1981.)*

powerless to make choices of how, when, where, and perhaps most importantly what they will dance. To feel out of control is a sure way to lose touch with the desire to dance.

Christine Spizzo (see profile, page 204) found that resigning from ABT was a liberating experience. As a guest artist with Ballet Arizona, Santa Fe Chamber Music Festival, Cynthia Gregory and Company, and other companies, she is rediscovering in her late thirties why it is that she first wanted to be a dancer:

> Dancing with the Arizona company was so stimulating and artistically satisfying. There were principal dancers from France, Italy, Spain, Switzerland, and New York. The choreographer, Jean-Paul Comelin, created movement for all of the different body types and styles, and allowed their individuality to flourish. . . . The pressures of free-lancing are so different. Self-sufficiency, and the ability to handle *everything* yourself, is the key. Standards of excellence are really self-imposed.

Staying in touch with what one really wants seems to be the key to longevity, whether one is age seventeen or seventy-seven. It is true, as dance writer Tobi Tobias argues, that the "athletic requirements of classical and most modern-dance techniques call for bodies in their prime, and the bloom of youth adds a sensual attraction to which viewers respond instinctively. [But witness Liz Lerman who] doesn't so much deny this conventional thinking as refuse to be limited by it."[3]

How to Dance?

In a highly provocative article that appeared in *Interchange,* Laban Movement Analyst and former modern dancer Carol-Lynne Moore argued that worldviews often rest upon contrasting "body metaphors."[4] Using body metaphors, dancers identify themselves with a figure of speech, not just an image. A simple example would be a thin dancer referring to himself as a "beanpole"; what is implied is *"I'm as skinny as* (a beanpole)." Dancers are familiar with the concept of body image; they should recognize that the concept of body metaphor is just as powerful in binding them to destructive training.

Of the four metaphors Moore discusses, the first two are the most destructive: the body as beast and the body as objet d'art. Each implies training paradigms that are common in dance. The remaining metaphors, the body as machine and the body as child, are less common in dance training but need to receive more attention by dance teachers.

The body-as-beast metaphor suggests that the body's willful spirit must be broken. The body is meant to be worked hard. In training, the emphasis is on repetition until the student "gets it right." Instruction based on this metaphor can be harmful. The student may tire while repeating the movement (e.g., a series of jumps) and make harmful compensations to complete the specified number of jumps in the time allotted (e.g., repeatedly landing on half-toe without allowing the heel to come in contact with the floor).

The body-as-objet d'art metaphor regards the body as an artistic object: the normative beauty of that object is established by each culture and era. In some dance, the standards have changed little—the rigidly erect posture and turned-out presentational stance of the courtier are here to stay in ballet. Emphasis on this metaphor is problematic. The visual aspect—how a position *looks*—is overemphasized in a kinetic art form. But it's not enough to strike a position and look good in it; the appearance must be dynamically maintained. The flexibility and strength must be dynamic and functional—something for which dancers must train.

The body-as-machine metaphor implies that the body is a well-designed, finely honed instrument; it is a fine-tuned engine. Once the machine is programmed, it is difficult to change: the well-trained ballerina may learn to dance a modern piece, but have great difficulties making changes in later rehearsals. To some degree, the metaphor may be appropriate. After all, consuming appropriate fuels for the body (complex carbohydrates) and applying biomechanical principles of movement allow dancers to use the "instrument" to the fullest. Such training information is important as long as dancers realize that the science of movement supports—not replaces—the art of dance.

The body-as-child metaphor emphasizes the developmental, inquiring, and creative nature of dance training. The instructor is there to stimulate, guide, and nurture the student. As long as the dancer maintains an active role in this guided self-discovery, this is clearly the teaching paradigm of choice.

Dancers who have studied with various instructors have thought of their bodies in all of these ways, to varying degrees. Whatever the metaphor of choice, dancers should find a worldview of teaching and training that makes sense to them. They must develop an informational base that is a protective shield against harmful training and destructive teachers.

The search is a lifetime process and the information does not come easily, but with this "body wisdom" comes a heightened sense of self-preservation and survival. Dancers can then take certain kinds of risks and not others, questioning what is being asked of them in training, following paradigms that are based on both the art and science of dance.

What to Dance?

To dance safely and sanely is not to throw away virtuosity. Choreography can be exciting without being dangerous, but some choreography is clearly dangerous to perform. Dancers must assess for themselves whether or not material is appropriate for their bodies. Questioning choreographic material will not make dancers popular with artistic directors—taking control of one's own life never will.

Dancing for Others

Who is going to stop and ask "Is it safe?" when dancing someone else's choreography? Although some female principals at NYCB can decide whether or not to perform particular steps in a ballet, NYCB female ensemble members know that there are dozens of dancers waiting to fill their pointe shoes. Among leading modern dance companies, the situation is not much better. Mark Morris's choreography, for example, can be compelling, but it takes its toll on the dancers. Yet when a company is small, who can afford to lobby for less-abusive choreography?

However, young dancers must realize that being passive and quiet isn't going to get them very far anyway. Only a very small percentage of dancers reach prima ballerina, premier danseur, or favored soloist status in classical and modern dance companies, and of those who do, a number don't last long.

Dancers have to recognize their limitations and reflect on what is being asked of them. Former NYCB-principal Patricia McBride recalls, "I wasn't like Allegra Kent, who could bend herself into a pretzel. I *was* unique however in my energy and love of dance." It is that love of dance that engages an audience more than the mere height of an extension or a perfect split-leap en l'air.

Jerel Hilding (Fig. 40), who recently retired from the Joffrey Ballet, admits, "I will not push; I will not force myself into some [position] which is unnatural. This may have inhibited my career, since I would not force certain positions, but it was never an obsession anyway."

Dancing Your Own Choreography

Dancers who feel the need to perform their own choreography have already begun to take control of their lives. This sentiment is echoed by Wendy Perron:

> When the material that you're dancing is your own choreography, you increase your longevity. For a while I couldn't jump because landing was so painful for my knees. I worked on my legs, adding ankle weights to my morning regimen in order to strengthen certain muscles. I still keep away from a lot of jumping or fast squats because I want my knees to last as long as possible. So there's a certain allowance in my own choreography—and also a certain authority that comes with maturity.

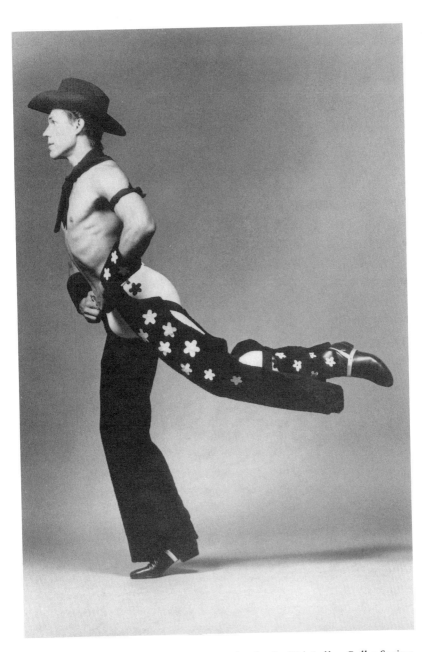

Figure 40. Jerel Hilding in the title role of *Billy the Kid,* Joffrey Ballet Spring Season 1988. Hilding admits the irony of having gotten this choice role, just as he retired from the company. *(Photo by Herbert Migdoll. Courtesy of the Joffrey Ballet.)*

Dancers who choreograph are able to exploit their own talents without compromising their health. Their focus obviously is more on what is being communicated than what movements can be substituted for leaps. Carmen de Lavallade (Fig. 41) offers:

> You must take stock of where you are physically. I can throw my legs over my head—I've done all that stuff. I don't have to do it all over again now. When you're older you have reached that height of performing and presence and experience. You don't have to do ten pirouettes to prove anything. There are thousands of ways to say something. When the body is older and wiser, you can say the same thing without all that show. It takes a lifetime to learn even how to stand on the stage.

As the dancers mature and continue to choreograph and perform, it is apparent that what is being said is more profound than how it is being said. Ten pirouettes may or may not be profound; standing on the stage and lifting an arm may or may not be profound. There are many ways to make a statement, but first one needs a statement to make. If dancers have nothing to say at age thirty, they're not going to start talking when they're sixty.

These days, however, dance has been popularized to a point that major touring companies—ballet, modern, jazz, ethnic—are giving audiences the "razzle-dazzle" they want to see, with the focus on the technical expertise of the dancer rather than on the dance. Thus, for example, the Bolshoi Ballet tours with little packages of second acts, flashy highlights taken out of time and out of place. (The integrity of an entire modern dance piece is more difficult to compromise.) There's little for the audiences to have to understand and that's the way they like it. This is how ballets suffer aesthetically and become little more than exhibits of athletically skilled dancers—dance pyrotechnics, or rather dance pornography. In fact, dancers should be fully integrated with the work, *become* it, in order to "exist wholly within the dynamic illusion of the dance."[5]

There is no doubt that dance aesthetics must be reconsidered. Audiences must bring more than passive receptivity to the dance and be more generous in what and whom they are willing to see on stage. This is a tall order for most dance audiences—dancers know it and so do artistic directors.

Bruce Marks, former principal dancer with ABT and currently artistic director of the Boston Ballet, says, "It's true I sometimes get comments from the audience about some of my larger dancers. But I

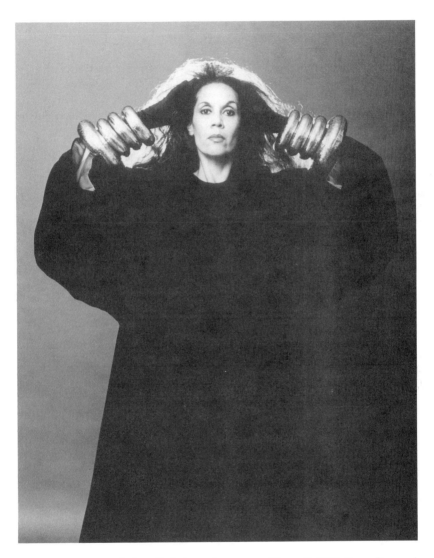

Figure 41. Carmen de Lavallade in performance. *(Photo © 1991 Kenn Duncan)*

don't pay attention." Let's hope that dancers and other artistic directors will follow suit.

What Earnings and Working Conditions?

No one goes into dance for the money. Nevertheless, there may be more money to be made in dance than dancers think.

When freelance writer Gloria Byron wrote an article, "Making Money Talk," for *Dance Magazine,* she called the topic "the touchiest of issues."[6] Why is talk of money a touchy issue? She suggests, "Tradition has long held that an individual's income is nobody's business but his or her own."[7] How convenient for the money interests in dance. Imperfect information means imperfect decisions, especially for dancers making effective money demands.

The distribution of income in dance is tremendously skewed. The Mikhail Baryshnikovs, Rudolf Nureyevs, Cynthia Gregorys, and Fernando Bujoneses enjoy a six- or seven-digit annual income (including perfume sales, manufacturers' ad revenues, and film contracts). On the other hand, at the time of this writing, a first-year dancer with The Joffrey Ballet would make 500 to 600 dollars a week for forty weeks, with health insurance and pension benefits. Most dancers in small, community-based companies would receive little to no remuneration for rehearsal and performance.

Those who try to produce their own dance—direct a company, choreograph, perform, and raise money—have an especially difficult time. Rehearsal spaces are few. Performance spaces are limited and expensive. Financing performance spaces and fund-raising for technical support and dancers' salaries is a full-time job. As a recent article expressed it, "America must think that the only good artist is a starving artist. . . . Aside from the energy and concentration needed to imagine new dances, presenting a concert requires the penurious cunning of old Scrooge himself."[8]

The good news is that—at least for some companies—incomes are on the rise. At NYCB, which like other New York–based companies has its own contract with the American Guild of Musical Artists (AGMA) that is separate from the National Basic Dance Agreement, a fifth-year corps de ballet dancer in the 1988–89 season earned a minimum base salary of 855 dollars a week for a guaranteed minimum of thirty-eight weeks. This is more than its top principals earned twelve years ago.[9]

Protecting Dancers' Rights: The Dancers' Union

Formed over fifty years ago to provide the performing artist with "sustenance and protection,"[10] AGMA has more than 6,000 members, including dancers, chorus singers, solo singers, opera stage directors, choreographers, and stage managers and assistants. AGMA maintains contact with company delegates to monitor work conditions. In recent years, they have negotiated for supplemental disability insurance, severance pay, dental plans, vacation pay, improved touring conditions, flooring specifications, appropriate theatre temperatures, and even changes in unsafe choreography and inappropriate costuming (like the nude, or partly nude, ballet that was cancelled because the bareskinned, perspiring dancers would suffer friction burns).

AGMA membership provides access to the AGMA Relief Fund, "a financial safety net for members who are aged, sick, disabled, and unable to meet obligations for medical care or essential living expenses."[11]

Most major companies—including NYCB, ABT, The Joffrey Ballet, San Francisco Ballet, Boston Ballet—are members of AGMA. Dancers pay 526 dollars to join (500 dollars initiation fee; 26 dollars basic dues) if their initial contract is for 2,000 dollars or more. Suzanne Gordon, in her book *Off Balance,* has convincingly characterized the rather passive union as anything but supportive of dancers.[12] However, many of the dancers I interviewed spoke favorably of the union, and in recent years it has effectively supported arbitration bids by dancers such as Christine Spizzo, Raymond Serrano, and Hilda Morales.[13]

Taking Action: ABT as a Case Study

The dance market is glutted with professional dancers, especially ballerinas, churned out nonstop by professional schools. Many of the dancers would *pay* for the privilege of dancing with a major professional company—dancers are clearly expendable. This becomes especially obvious when a company dancer grows too old, too injured, or too "unreliable," no matter how caring and nurturing the "family" was until then. When the submissive dancer becomes more assertive, conflict may result.

Clearly, dancers should consider their dance colleagues, directors, and administrators not as members of an extended family, but as members of two separate interests or classes—labor and management. Cora Cahan, executive director of Feld Ballets NY, has commented, "Dance people tend to be families, historically, so contracts and the formalization of relationships are relatively new. I would say that it's in the last fifteen years that we're beginning to see contracts."[14]

When ABT dancers, who were lower-paid than the musicians and stagehands in the theatre, wanted to negotiate more favorable contracts in 1979, the administration was not amused. The dancers had hired labor lawyer Leonard Leibowitz to represent them, in tandem with AGMA. The union paid one-quarter of his fee and the dancers paid the rest. The dancers had done their homework: they had examined the ABT Basic Agreement and surveyed the entire rank and file of the company to verify any special contract arrangements. They also obtained data on salaries and working conditions in other companies.

After weeks of negotiation, the dancers rejected a small salary and benefit increase offered by management. In turn, the company locked the dancers out of their studios and cancelled part of their winter season. The dancers began to speak out in public about the exploitation.

What was it that they wanted? They wanted an increase in salaries, something considerably more than the 5 percent over three years that ABT offered them. This 5 percent, costing about 150,000 dollars over three years for the seventy-seven dancers involved, was roughly the equivalent of the annual salary offered to Russian defector Alexander Godunov shortly thereafter.

They also demanded improved working conditions, such as adequate flooring and dry-cleaned costumes, advanced schedule notices, and an increase to at least forty in the number of weeks of guaranteed employment. The dancers were also interested in guarantees in severance pay, in better financial provisions for hotel and food allowances when touring, and supplemental unemployment benefits, not to mention pensions (which have yet to become standard in dance).[15]

Of particular importance was the creation of a job security clause. In 1982, this demand was successfully negotiated (along with additional gains in salary and working conditions). Procedures were established for dismissal. Dancers could no longer be dismissed without just cause or good and sufficient artistic reasons.

One of the key actors in these negotiations was ABT's Christine Spizzo (see profile on page 204). Despite the protracted and somewhat unpleasant negotiations, Spizzo is proud of her association with ABT—as a dedicated artist and as a union representative fighting for dancers' rights:

> [I am] an American dancer who has and is making a living in this country in classical ballet. In Europe, many ballet companies are state-supported and operated; that's not the case in the United States—although outside of the Coasts (New York and California) there is a much-improved quality of dancers' repertory. In the United States in general, though, dancers still have to fight for adequate salaries and decent working conditions. This is something we all must do. Dancing can be a *career* here, not just something you do when you're in your twenties.

Dancers like Spizzo show by example that all dancers can love dance and still make demands for better salaries and better working conditions. Dancers can and should be aggressive in their demands.

ABT's contract negotiations are not meant to serve as a blueprint for all dancers and all dance companies. Collective bargaining may not be an option for dancers in local dance groups, who are unhappy about poor working conditions, hard floors, or cold theatres. They are not as organized as "management." It may not be an option for dancers teaching jazz part-time at a university, who inevitably are scheduled for the worst hours. All they want is a little financial security to subsidize their choreographic pursuits.

Still, the empowerment process is clear, irrespective of idiom or work situation. Find information, compare, talk, communicate. It's a beginning, even though there are no guarantees of success.

In all aspects of dance, audiences must become more sympathetic and dancers more assertive, challenging damaging body metaphors, training regimens, dietary patterns, and company practices. If dance is about communication, dancers must now practice their verbal skills. They must share ideas that challenge the status quo to make changes happen in the dance world.

For most dancers, taking control of their life means that they demand to be treated with dignity and respect, that they emphasize their self-worth rather than self-sacrifice, that they find a balance between the passion and the reality of dance. To do any less is a disservice to the role models they emulated and promised to transcend and to the students whose role models they become. It is a sobering thought.

Photo © Johan Elbers, 1990

Wendy Perron

Wendy Perron has been teaching, choreographing, and performing for more than twenty years. She appeared with the Trisha Brown Company between 1975 and 1978 and currently directs the Wendy Perron Dance Company. She has toured throughout the United States, Canada, and Europe, and as a writer she has been published in *Dance Research Journal, Contact Quarterly, Ballet Review, Dance Magazine, The Drama Review,* and the *Village Voice.*

Perron believes it is her early injuries (to the upper back, knees, and ankles) twenty years ago that may have actually saved her. The injuries taught her about the limits of her body and what she had to do to work within them. For example, she knows that she must perform a daily regimen of stretches, ball work (kinetic awareness), and leg weights. She also knows that her key to longevity in dance is to perform her own choreography:

> I don't have to choreograph a lot of jumps or very fast squats into my movement. I don't need to dance kneeling on my knees. Even when I danced with Trisha Brown, I used knee pads for such movement. As I get older, I realize that there's a certain authority that comes with maturity—I don't have to arch my back to prove

anything; what I do have to do is keep the resilience in my movement. This is the key to injury prevention.

I have always gone for longevity in dance. After all, I am a dancer. That's what I do. I didn't want to reach seventy and stop dancing. But if the pleasure stopped, I would stop. If I wasn't enjoying it, I wouldn't do it. This is one of the reasons why I've lasted so long and others—for instance, some people I know who went to the Juilliard School—quit.

You have to keep the joy alive; to do this you have to recognize your limitations early on. I could have broken my body, but I didn't. At the Graham School, where I was on scholarship after graduation from Bennington, they wanted to discipline everyone the same way, but I was somewhat defiant; for example, I would not do the first bounces as fast as they wanted.

That defiance may have saved her as well. In her early forties, she is very much her own dancer, refusing to take class with anyone who superimposes a movement style injurious to her body. She continues to choreograph and perform. In some ways, she has just begun her creative explorations. Each year, her movement seems more fluid, playful, and unpredictable, appealing yet challenging.

For Perron, finding a balance in dance means balancing performance schedules, choreographing, obligations to family (she is a mother) and friends, writing, and organizing in the peace movement. If one can say no to beginning ballet class with a fifth position grand plié, one can probably say no to anything, which leaves a lot of room for everything else that's important in dance.

. . . .

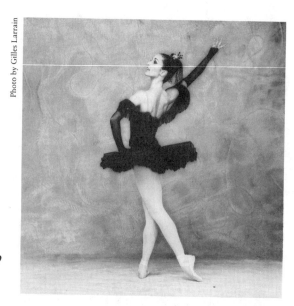

Photo by Gilles Larrain

Christine Spizzo

Christine Spizzo joined ABT in 1975 and danced for thirteen years with the company, the last eight as a featured soloist. Before joining ABT, she had had a taste of professional dance, performing with the National Ballet of Washington, D.C., and Ballet Repertory Company.

She enjoyed a number of interesting roles with ABT, including Calliope in *Apollo*, Amour in *Don Quixote*, the Pigtail Girl in *Graduation Ball*, Diamond in *Sleeping Beauty*, a Chinese dancer in *The Nutcracker*, the Youngest Sister in *Pillar of Fire*, the leading roles in the third movement of *Bourrée Fantastique* and the first movement of *Concerto*, and a featured role in *Airs*. It is perhaps this last dance, choreographed by Paul Taylor in 1978 and full of furious leaps and slides and hurling through the air, that caused her the most injuries over the years.

Airs requires pirouettes on the knees and drops in one count from standing to kneeling. The dancers dance barelegged and although they can use knee pads during rehearsal, that's not an option during performance. Spizzo, as a featured performer in the dance, racked up several injuries—quadriceps strains, microtears to the tendons of her kneecaps, and recurrent calf-muscle strains. A lot of this had to do with the running in plié that the dance requires, for which classical ballet dancers are not trained. More and more, she began questioning what she was asked to do in the repertory, and what she was *not* asked to do. Ultimately, she left the company.

Spizzo considers herself a dedicated artist as well as a committed union representative. Dance *can* be a career. She has been a guest artist with Ballet Arizona and other companies. She has completed a national tour of Nureyev and Friends. Her standard of living has increased together with her self-esteem.

Spizzo acknowledges that the norm in classical dance still favors younger dancers. It's perhaps just a little less blatant outside the big two or three New York–based ballet companies.

. . . .

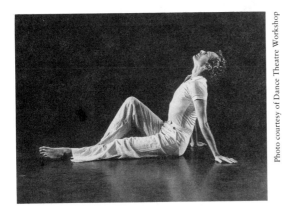

Photo courtesy of Dance Theatre Workshop

Jeff Duncan

Jeff Duncan had many lives, and he fought very hard to find a balance among all of them—teacher, choreographer, producer (he was a co-founder of New York's Dance Theatre Workshop, with Jack Moore and Art Bauman), and designer. He delighted in crafting his choreography, serious, dramatic, and dark though it was. He delighted in the jewelry he made, in the dance he produced, in the artists he organized.

He didn't delight as much in the young dancers he taught, who were more interested in dieting, diuretics, and développé than in varying the intensity with which one could perform even the simplest movements. He would try their patience mightily just by spending half a class working on "scallops"—semicircles in alternating directions that swept across the floor.

For Duncan, this was what technique was all about: performing simple movements, taking risks and making mistakes, consuming as much of the floor space as possible, moving without deliberating, moving as if one's life depended on it, with urgency and with joy. The impetus for the movement, the emotional impetus, was what would determine whether or not a movement sequence would be successful. This is what he himself had been taught by Hanya Holm, Doris Humphrey, Anna Sokolow, and others.

He was always trying to make his students critical consumers of all the dance styles they studied. He questioned the "why" of a particular movement and invited his students to do the same. If they didn't believe him in class—that technique was learned and developed through the simplest of movements—many of them became "believers" when they saw him perform in some of his powerful works like *Antique Epigrams* or *Oracle* or *Canticle*. After all, watching masters in performance is perhaps the best way to demonstrate technique.

Another victim of AIDS, Jeff Duncan died in May 1989 at the age of fifty-nine. At the time he was still organizing and trying to produce dance in Baltimore, and trying to motivate some of those younger dancers to care enough to do more and be more than they ever thought possible. How? By working on those simple "scallops" that demanded every bit of training and focus a dancer could recall and give.

Directory of Selected Dance/ Arts Medicine Clinics

Adapted from work by Jan Dunn. Copyright © 1990 Jan Dunn.

West

California

Long Beach Sports Medicine and Physical Therapy Center, Inc.
2017 Palo Verde Ave., Suite 101
Long Beach, CA 90815
(213) 493-5501
Staff: Dan Bailey, R.P.T.; George J. Walter, R.P.T.

The Los Angeles Dance Clinic
10921 Wilshire Blvd., #LL–7
Los Angeles, CA 90024
(213) 824-9723
Staff: Daniel M. Silver, M.D.; Rene Muhlenkamp, R.P.T.

Sports Medicine Associates
1835 South Sepulveda Blvd.
West Los Angeles, CA 90025
(213) 477-6950
Staff: Michael Schreiber, D.O.

Center for Sports Medicine
Dance Medicine Division

St. Francis Memorial Hospital
900 Hyde St.
San Francisco, CA 94109
(415) 775-4321
Staff: James Garrick, M.D.; Patrice L. Whiteside, M.A.; Elizabeth J. Larkin,
    M.A.; Chris Fittsimmons, R.P.T.

Health Program for Performing Artists
San Francisco Medical Center
University of California
400 Parnassus Ave., 5th floor
Box 0326
San Francisco, CA 94143
(415) 476-7373

Bresler Center Medical Group
2901 Wilshire Blvd., #345
Santa Monica, CA 90403
(213) 828-6471
Staff: David Bresler, Ph.D.

Santa Monica Orthopedic
1301 20th St., Suite 150
Santa Monica, CA 90404
(213) 829-2663
Staff: Bert Mandelbaum, M.D.

Colorado

University of Colorado Health Sciences Center
Department of Neurology
Campus Box B–183
4200 E. 9th Ave.
Denver, CO 80262
(303) 270-7566
Staff: Stuart Schneck, M.D.

Northwest

Washington

Seattle Sports Medicine
501 First Avenue South
Seattle, WA 98104
(206) 467-6705

Staff: John W. Robertson, M.D.; Karen Clippinger-Robertson, M.S.P.E.; Ken Foreman, Ph.D.; Boyd Bender, P.T.

University of Washington Sports Medicine Clinic
242 Hec Edmundson Pavillion, GB–15
Seattle, WA 98195
(206) 543-1552
Staff: Carol C. Teitz, M.D. (for dancers); several additional medical staff members

Southwest

Texas

Arts Medicine Center
Austin Regional Clinic
P.O. Box 26726
Austin, TX 78755-0726
(512) 343-6268 (center)
(512) 458-4276 (clinic)
Staff: Stephen A. Mitchell, M.D. (director)

Performing Arts Clinic
University of Texas Health Science Center
Houston, TX 77030
(713) 792-5777
Staff: Alan Lockwood, M.D. (director)

Midwest

Illinois

Chicago Sports Medicine Dance Injury Center
25 E. Washington St.
Chicago, IL 60602
(312) 332-6570
Staff: David A. Birnbaum, M.D. (director)

Medical Program for Performing Artists of the Rehabilitation Institute of Chicago
Rehabilitation Institute of Chicago
345 E. Superior St.
Chicago, IL 60611
(312) 908-ARTS
Staff: Alice Brandfonbrenner, M.D. (director)

Indiana

Performing Arts Medicine Program
Indiana University School of Medicine
541 Clinical Dr.
Indianapolis, IN 46202
(317) 274-4225
Staff: Kenneth D. Brandt, M.D. (director)

Ohio

Center for Orthopedic Care
2123 Auburn Ave., Suite 235
Cincinnati, OH 45219
(513) 651-0094
Staff: G. James Sammarco, M.D. (director)

Cleveland Clinic Foundation
Medical Center for Performing Arts
9500 Euclid Ave.
Cleveland, OH 44195
(216) 444-5545
Staff: Richard Lederman, M.D. (director)

South

Kentucky

Louisville Performing Arts Center for Health (PACH)
Department of Psychiatry
University of Louisville
Louisville, KY 40292
(502) 588-1936
Staff: Judith R. F. Kupersmith, M.D. (director)

North Carolina

Capital Physical Therapy, Inc.
6164 Falls of the Neuse
Raleigh, NC 27609
(919) 467-0030
Staff: Cathy E. Busby, M.S., P.T.

Department of Orthopedic Surgery
Duke University Medical Center
Durham, NC 27710
(919) 684-4007

Staff: William T. Hardaker, Jr., M.D.; William E. Garrett, M.D., Ph.D.; Robert Bartlett, M.D. (chairman, Department of Physical Therapy)

Northeast

Massachusetts

Boston Arts Medicine
1330 Beacon St.
Brookline, MA 02146
(617) 232-6646
Staff: Richard N. Norris, M.D. (director)

Musical Medicine Clinic
1 Hawthorne Place, Suite 103
Boston, MA 02114
(617) 726-8657
Staff: Fred Hochberg, M.D. (director)

New York

The Center for Dance Medicine
41 E. 42nd St., #200
New York, NY 10017
(212) 685-8113
Staff: Richard Bachrach, D.O.; Irene Dowd; Mavis Lockwood

Department of Orthopedic Surgery
Hospital for Joint Diseases Orthopedic Institute
301 E. 17th St.
New York, NY 10003
(212) 598-6497
Staff: Victor Frankel, M.D. (director)

East Side Sports Physical Therapy
244 E. 84th St.
New York, NY 10028
(212) 570-0209
Staff: Anthony J. Saraniti, M.S., P.T.

Harkness Center for Dance Injuries at the Hospital for Joint Diseases
301 E. 17th St.
New York, NY 10003
(212) 598-6022
Staff: Mindy Forman, P.T.

Kathryn and Gilbert Miller
Health Care Institute for Performing Arts
425 W. 59th St., Room 6A
New York, NY 10019
(212) 523-6200
Staff: Emil Pascarelli, M.D. (director)

Lenox Hill Hospital
Institute of Sports Medicine and Athletic Trauma
130 E. 77th St.
New York, NY 10021
(212) 439-2345
Staff: James A. Nicholas, M.D. (director); George Veras (assistant director);
    Marijeanne Liederbach, M.S., A.T.C. (research assistant)

Performing Arts Center for Health (PACH)
Mental Hygiene Clinic
Bellevue Hospital
400 E. 30th St.
New York, NY 10016
(212) 561-4073; messages (212) 561-4711
Staff: Howard W. Telson, M.D. (director)

Performing Center for Health
(Medical/psychiatric referral service for artists)
(212) 247-1560
Contact: Marian Horosko

West Side Dance Physical Therapy
2109 Broadway, Suite 204
New York, NY 10023
(212) 787-0397
Staff: Marika E. Molnar, M.S., P.T.

West Side Sports Physical Therapy
2109 Broadway, Suite 204
New York, NY 10023
(212) 799-0160
Staff: Charlotte J. Coren, M.S., P.T.

Pennsylvania

The Medical Center for Performing Arts
Suburban General Hospital
2705 DeKalb Pike
Norristown, PA 19401
(215) 279-1060
Staff: David Rosenfeld, M.D.

The Arts Medicine Center
Thomas Jefferson University Hospital
11th and Walnut Sts.
Philadelphia, PA 19107
(215) 955-8300

Glossaries

Dance

à la seconde.   A position or movement in which one leg is extended directly to the side of the body, either with the toe touching the floor or with the leg lifted to various heights.

adagio.   A slow, sustained tempo in a particular movement; section of a ballet class; pas de deux. Adagio movements are characterized by continuity, fluidity, and apparent ease of execution.

allegro.   A fast, lively tempo or movement characterized by a quality of lightness, quickness, and buoyancy. Allegro also refers to a section of a ballet class.

arabesque.   A pose or movement in which one leg is raised directly behind the body. The supporting leg may be fully extended, flexed, or on pointe, but the raised leg must be fully extended. If the raised leg is bent, the position or movement is called attitude derrière.

attitude turns.   Turns on one leg in which the other leg is lifted either to the front, to the side, or to the back. The knee of the lifted leg is bent, usually at a 90-degree angle. As in arabesque, the supporting leg may be fully extended, flexed, or on demi- or full-pointe.

barre.   The railing used to provide support for dancers during specific exercises in a dance class; a specific section of a dance class. The barre section of a dance class features exercises that build strength and agility of particular muscle groups. In a center barre, such exercises are performed away from and without the support of the barre; in a floor barre, they are performed while lying on the floor.

batterie. Steps in which the legs beat together in a scissorlike motion. Petite batterie are small-beat steps, such as brisés and entrechats, that demand precision and quickness. Grande batterie are large-beat steps, such as cabrioles and grands jetés en tournant battus, that require elevation and strength.

brisé. A small beating step that travels. Brisé begins by brushing the working leg away from the supporting leg, beating the legs together in the air, and landing on either one or both legs.

cabriole. An elevation step in which the stretched legs beat in the air.

classical ballet. Ballet based on the danse d'école or codified theatrical dance principles.

corps, corps de ballet. Group or ensemble members of a dance or ballet company.

courtier. A member of the royal court.

danseur noble. A leading male dancer who embodies classical ballet style.

demi-plié. See **plié.**

demi-pointe ("half-pointe," "half-toe") Balancing or moving on the balls of the feet.

développé. A folding, then unfolding or extension, of one leg in any direction.

en croix ("in the shape of a cross") A pattern of repetition in which an action is performed to the front, to the side, and then to the back in sequence.

en l'air ("in the air") Any action or movement in which either one or both legs leave the ground, as in tour en l'air (*q.v.*) or rond de jambe en l'air (see **rond de jambe**).

entrechat. A beating step in which the legs cross and uncross a certain number of times.

ethnic dance. Dance of a specific region or culture.

fifth position. A closed position of the feet in which the legs are turned out from the hip and the heel of the front foot is placed at the big toe joint of the foot behind.

first position. A closed position of the feet in which the legs are turned out from the hip with both heels close together and the toes pointing away from the midline of the body.

fondu. A flexion or bending of the supporting leg.

Graham contraction. A stylized abdominal contraction with the head falling backward in hyperextension and the arms reaching forward with wrists hyperextended; basic to the technique developed by Martha Graham.

grand allegro. A section of a ballet or class that combines large jumps, batterie, and turns. It is usually one of the final combinations of a ballet class.

grand battement ("large beat") A large kick in which the working leg is forcefully raised, then lowered with control, in any direction.

grand jeté ("large leap") A leap or jeté is an active transfer of weight from one foot to the other in which both feet leave the floor. A grand jeté is a forceful spring from one foot to the other in which the gesturing or unsupported leg is thrust into the direction of the leap.

grand plié. See **plié.**

grande batterie. See **batterie.**

modern dance. A term used to indicate dance or styles of dance arising in the twentieth century and not based in classical ballet technique.

pas. A simple step or movement that involves a transfer of weight.

pas de deux. A dance or series of steps performed by two people; a duet.

pathogenic choreography. Movements or sequences that are potentially hazardous owing to extreme physical stresses or demands placed on the body.

petite batterie ("small beats") See **batterie.**

pirouette. A turn of the body on one leg.

plié. A flexion or bending of one or both legs: demi-, partial; grande, full.

pointe, sur les pointes. Balancing or moving on the tips of the toes, usually with the support of a blocked shoe.

premier danseur. A leading male ballet dancer.

relevé. Raising the body through plantar flexion ("extending" the foot while maintaining contact with the floor) of either one or both ankles.

rond de jambe. A circling action of the whole leg, executed with the foot leading either away from the body (en dehors) or toward the body (en dedans). Rond de jambe may be performed with the toe maintaining contact with the floor (à terre) or with the toe off the floor (en l'air).

show dance. Theatrical dance styles used in musicals, revues, and music videos. Show dance often combines characteristics of jazz, tap, and ballet.

soloist. A solo dancer.

tendu. Pointing the foot and stretching the leg continuously in a particular direction (e.g., behind the body—tendu derrière), with the toe maintaining contact with the floor.

tour en l'air. A turn in the air that usually starts in fifth position demi-plié and returns to fifth or an open position. During the turn, the body is held vertically and the legs are held tightly together.

tour jeté, grand jeté en tournant entrelacé, grand jeté dessus en tournant.   A large turning leap in which the legs pass closely together as the body changes direction in the air to finally land in an arabesque.

turnout.   External rotation of the entire leg, most of which occurs at the hip.

unitard.   A type of dance apparel that combines the traditional tights and leotard of ballet into a sleek, one-piece garment.

Medical and Technical

abduction.   Movement of an extremity or limb segment away from the midline of the body.

abductors.   Muscles that move the extremities or limb segments away from the midline of the body.

acetabulum.   The cup-shaped depression of the pelvis that constitutes the socket for the head of the femur. The acetabulum is also commonly called the "hip socket."

Achilles tendon.   The tendon that connects the calcaneous (the heel bone) to the muscles of the calf (gastrocnemius, soleus, and plantaris).

acromion process.   The outside edge of the spine of the scapula; it articulates with the clavicle (collarbone).

acupuncturist.   A healer trained in strategic placing of thin needles in the muscles of the body to relieve pain and effect cure.

adduction.   Movement of an extremity or limb segment toward or beyond the midline of the body.

adductors.   Muscles that move the extremities or limb segments toward the midline of the body.

aerobic activity.   Continuous and relatively moderate exercise that is at least twelve to fifteen minutes in duration.

anaerobic ("without oxygen") Refers to energy systems in which heat energy is ultimately generated in the absence of oxygen, usually through relatively short workouts.

angle of femoral anteversion.   The angle created by the neck of the femur and the shaft of the femur in the transverse plane, which is affected by the amount of torsion or rotation intrinsic to the femur or hip. With a high angle of anteversion (greater than 12 degrees), the femur is rotated to the front, making turnout of the leg difficult. With a low angle (less than 12 degrees, called retroversion [*q.v.*]), the femur has a more posterior rotation, making turnout of the leg easier.

anorexia nervosa. An eating disorder characterized by severe emaciation resulting from self-imposed weight loss.

anterior. Refers to the front side of the body.

anterior deltoid. A cap-shaped muscular formation covering the anterior portion of the shoulder joint.

anterior hip capsule. The front portion of the hip capsule.

anterior pelvic tilt. A forward tilt of the pelvis that increases the curve of the lumbar spine (hyperextension).

arthritis. Inflammation of a joint.

arthroscope. An instrument that is equipped with a light and camera for viewing inside a joint during surgery.

arthroscopy. Surgery on the interior of a joint using an arthroscope. May also be used for diagnosis of disorders.

ballistic stretch. A stretch that involves rapid bouncing, lunging, or bobbing.

biceps brachii. A two-headed muscle of the anterior portion of the upper arm.

biomechanics. The study of the principles and laws of mechanics applied to the function of human movement, usually using quantitative data.

body therapist. A practitioner trained in a body-therapy approach (e.g., Bartenieff Fundamentals, Feldenkrais, Ideokinesis) to movement rehabilitation.

bulimia. An eating disorder characterized by compulsive eating, usually followed by self-induced vomiting.

bunion. A deformity of the first metatarsal phalangeal joint, characterized by an enlarged bump at the inside of the big-toe joint.

bursa. A fluid-filled sac.

bursitis. Inflammation of a bursa.

carpals. Bones of the wrist.

cartilage. The nonvascular connective tissue that interfaces between the bones of the joint.

cathartics. Medications that increase the rate of bowel evacuation.

chiropractor. A licensed, certified practitioner who manipulates neuromuscular structures of the body to restore and maintain their proper functioning.

cinematography, cinematographic analysis. The use of film to analyze movement.

clavicle. The collarbone. This bone articulates with the sternum (the breastbone) and the acromion process of the scapula.

coccyx. The tailbone, or last three to five vertebrae of the spine.

collagen. The major protein of connective tissue, cartilage, and bone.

compression fracture. A break—usually in bone or cartilage—caused by increased pressure from external forces.

concentric contraction. A contraction of the muscle fibers that causes the muscle to shorten.

coracobrachialis. A muscle that originates in the coracoid process of the scapula and inserts in the medial border of the humerus.

cortisone. A steroidal medication used to decrease inflammation.

crepitus. Noise within a joint.

deltoid muscle. A triangular-shaped muscle of the shoulder that connects the clavicle and scapula to the humerus.

diaphragm muscle. A muscular membrane that separates the abdominal cavity from the thoracic cavity.

dietician. A practitioner who examines the relationship of diet to health for the maintenance of health and prevention of disease.

distal. An extremity or limb segment situated away from the center of the body.

diuretics. Substances that promote urination, thus decreasing fluid retention.

dorsiflexion or **ankle flexion.** Bending action of the ankle or foot joints that causes the top of the foot or toes to come closer to the shin.

eccentric contraction. A contraction of the muscle that causes the muscle to lengthen against resistance.

electromyography. A method of testing muscle action: electrodes are inserted into specific muscles and the electrical action potentials of the muscles are recorded and analyzed.

emetics. Agents that promote vomiting.

erector spinae. Muscles of the back that hold the spine erect.

eversion. Raising the lateral border of the foot so that the foot rests mostly on its inner edge. Also a component of rolling in (*q.v.*) and winging (*q.v.*) the foot.

extension. Extending a limb or body part; increasing the angle at a joint, such as straightening a knee.

external, outward, or **lateral rotation.** Turning or movement of a joint in the transverse plane, away from the midline of the body.

fascial sheath. A covering of connective tissue that envelops a muscle.

femur. The thigh bone.

flexion. Decreasing the angle at a joint, such as bending an elbow.

frontal plane. The plane that runs through the body from side to side and separates the front of the body from the back. Actions such as abduction and adduction occur in the frontal plane.

functional flexibility. The range of motion actually used during dance movements.

gastrocnemius. The large calf muscle that assists in plantar flexion—pointing the toe, relevé, or pushing off the ground (jumping).

general practitioner. A physician trained to take care of a broad range of medical conditions such as common illnesses, minor injuries, and trauma; a family physician.

glenohumeral adductors. Adductors of the glenohumeral (shoulder) joint, including pectoralis major, latissimus dorsi, teres major, and coracobrachialis.

gluteus maximus. The largest of the three gluteal muscles located in the buttocks. Gluteus maximus acts as a hip extensor in forceful movements.

goniometer. A device that measures the angle between different body segments.

groin. The junction of the thigh and the trunk.

hamstrings. A group of muscles in the back of the thigh that cross both the hip and the knee.

healer. A person who claims to heal by a specific method, system, or philosophy, such as Christian Science, "new thought," and laying on of hands. More generally, the term refers to an individual who has been trained in one of a number of culturally conventional and nonconventional healing practices.

heel lifts. Noncompressible pads placed inside one or both shoes.

herniated disc. A condition that occurs when the integrity of the outer fibrous covering of the disc—the anulus fibrosis—becomes weakened and the internal gelatinous body of the disc—the nucleus pulposus—projects through the covering. This causes compression on adjacent structures, nerves, and connective tissue.

high instep. A high-arched foot; a bony-appearing area just in front of the ankle, mostly common in highly arched feet.

homeopath. A practitioner of the system of therapy developed by Samuel Hahnemann, which treats disorders using minute doses of medication that, in healthy persons, would produce symptoms of the disorder.

humerus. The long bone of the upper arm.

hyperextension. Extreme extension; an increase of the angle between two joints to greater than 180 degrees.

ibuprofen. A nonsteroidal anti-inflammatory medication used in the management of pain and inflammation. Previously available only by prescription, it is now an over-the-counter medication.

iliofemoral ligament (" 'Y' ligament") A triangular ligament that connects the anterior inferior spine of the ilium, the rim of the acetabulum, and the femur. It inhibits hyperextension of the hip joint.

iliopsoas. A major hip flexor. Iliacus and psoas major comprise the iliopsoas. Psoas major originates on the vertebral bodies of the twelfth thoracic to the fifth lumbar vertebrae. Iliacus originates on the iliac crest and fossa. Both join and attach at the lesser trochanter of the femur.

internal, or **medial** or **inward, rotation.** Turning or movement of a joint in the transverse plane toward the midline of the body.

internist. A physician who specializes in the diagnosis and treatment of nonsurgical diseases, especially in adults.

intra-abdominal pressure. Pressure within the abdominal cavity created by the tonus of abdominal muscles. Muscles of the pelvic floor and diaphragm assist in influencing intra-abdominal pressure. This pressure helps to support internal organs and structures.

inversion. Raising the medial or inside border of the foot so that the foot rests mostly on its outer edge. Also a component of rolling out (*q.v.*) and sickling (*q.v.*).

inward rotators. Muscles that effect movement toward the midline of the body in the transverse plane.

ischial tuberosities. The "sit bones"; the lowest bony protrusions of the ischium.

ischium. One of the three bones that comprise the os coxa. The ischium is the lowest part of the pelvis.

isometric contraction. A muscular contraction in which there is no change in muscle length.

ketosis. Metabolic adaptation in which the body converts fatty acids and amino acids into ketone bodies (metabolized as carbohydrate substitutes). This allows the body to survive for extended periods of time without external sources of glucose.

kilocalorie ("Calorie") The amount of heat required to raise the temperature of one kilogram of water by 1° Celsius.

kinesiologist. A practitioner trained in the science and study of movement and the structures of the body involved in movement.

kinesiology. The qualitative and quantitative analysis of human movement as it relates to the neuromuscular system.

kinesthetic; kinesthesia. The sensation of body movement, position, and tension perceived by the nerves, muscles, tendons, and joints.

lactic acid. A metabolic by-product of strenuous muscular exertion.

lateral. Away from the midline of the body, for example, the outer side of the arms and legs.

latissimus dorsi. Broad muscle of the back and upper arm that originates on the spinous processes of the lower thoracic and lumbar vertebrae, the sacrum, the iliac crest, and the lower three or four ribs.

lever. A rigid body or object, such as a bone, that rotates around a fulcrum or axis. Levers operate on the principle that a force applied to one end of the lever will cause the other end to move in a direction opposite to the force applied.

ligaments. Sheets or bands of tissue that connect bones and limit the end-range of motion.

longitudinal arch. The arch on the underside of the foot that runs from the heel to the base of the toes.

lumbar compression. Compression of the lumbar region of the spine, most stressful when landing from a jump or lifting a heavy object.

lumbar intervertebral discs. The discs located between the lumbar vertebrae.

massage therapist. A practitioner who uses massage for the treatment or amelioration of specific neuromuscular or soft tissue problems.

medial. Toward or near the midline of the body, for example, the inner edge of the knee or ankle.

menisci, lateral and **medial** (sing., meniscus). Crescent-shaped cartilaginous structures located in the knee joint.

metacarpals. The five bones of the hand located just proximal to each finger.

metatarsals. The five bones of the foot located just proximal to each toe.

moment arm. The perpendicular distance between the line of force application and the axis of a lever.

neurologist. A physician who specializes in the treatment of neurological disorders.

neuromuscular patterning. The patterning of motor innervation of skeletal muscles.

neurovascular. Refers to arteries, veins, and nerves.

nutritionist. A practitioner trained in the study of food and drink needs of human beings for health or prevention of illness.

obliques, internal and **external.** Lateral abdominal muscles that contribute to intra-abdominal pressure.

orthopedist. A physician trained in the medical, surgical, and physical methods required for the diagnosis and treatment of skeletal system disorders.

os trigonum. A small triangular bone, sometimes present as part of the ankle (talus) bone.

osteopath. A practitioner trained in specific manipulative measures in addition to the normative diagnostic and therapeutic measures of medicine.

outward rotators Muscles that effect movement away from the midline of the body in the transverse plane.

paravertebral. Alongside the vertebrae or the spine.

patella. The knee cap.

patella chondromalacia. Softening (wear or tear) of the cartilage on the underside of the knee cap.

pectoralis major. A muscle of the chest that originates at the clavicle, the manubrium, the body of the sternum, and the first through sixth ribs and attaches at the humerus.

peroneal tendinitis. Inflammation of the tendons on the outside of the leg.

peroneus longus and **brevis.** Two muscles of the lower leg: peroneus brevis originates on the fibula and attaches at the fifth metatarsal; peroneus longus originates on the upper and outer surfaces of the fibula and tibia and inserts behind the lateral malleolus and continues under the foot and attaches to the medial cuneiform and first metatarsal.

phalanges. Bones of the toes or fingers.

physical therapist. A practitioner trained in specific rehabilitation techniques, such as massage, ultrasound treatment, and electrical stimulation.

plantar fascia. The sheet of fibrous tissue that supports muscles of the sole of the foot.

plantar fasciitis. Ligament inflammation that causes pain in the sole or heel of the foot.

plantar flexion. Moving the plantar (sole) surface of the foot downward. Commonly called "pointing the toe" in dance.

podiatrist. A practitioner concerned with the diagnosis, treatment, and rehabilitation of injuries and diseases of the human foot and ankle and those structures above that are affected by their actions.

posterior. Refers to the back surface or rear portion of the body.

posterior pelvic tilt. A tilt of the pelvis that reduces the curve of the lower lumbar spine.

pronation. Of the foot: lifting the outside edge of the foot (also called "rolling in" [q.v.]). Of the forearm: inward rotation of the lower arm that turns the palm toward the body.

prone.   Lying face down.

Proprioceptive Neuromuscular Facilitation (PNF).   A stretching technique in which isometric contraction against resistance is followed by muscle relaxation and then static stretching to achieve increased range of motion.

proprioceptivity.   Sensitivity to stimuli arising from muscles, tendons, and other tissues; sense of feeling, of balance.

proximal.   An extremity or limb segment situated toward the center of the body.

psoas.   A muscle that flexes the hip and connects the lumbar spine to the femur. See also **iliopsoas.**

psychiatrist.   A physician who specializes in the diagnosis and treatment of mental diseases and disorders.

psychologist.   A licensed practitioner concerned with human mental and behavioral processes.

psychotherapist.   A psychiatrist or psychologist trained in the treatment of emotional, behavioral, personality, or psychiatric disorders. Verbal or nonverbal processes of communication, rather than chemical measures, may be used in treating clients.

quadriceps.   A group of four muscles of the upper thigh that extend the knee. The four parts of the quadriceps are rectus femoris, vastus lateralis, vastus intermedius, and vastus medialis.

renal toxicity.   Toxicity that affects normal kidney function.

retroversion.   A femoral angle of torsion less than 12 degrees. This condition facilitates external rotation of the lower extremity, especially during movement.

Rolfing practitioner.   One trained in the theories of Ida Rolf, which emphasize deep tissue manipulation.

rolling in.   Pronation or eversion of the foot; lifting the outside border of the foot off the ground.

rolling out.   Supination, or inversion, of the foot; lifting the inside border of the foot off the ground.

rotator cuff.   A group of four muscles (subscapularis, supraspinatus, infraspinatus, and teres minor) that help to maintain contact between the head of the humerus and the scapula.

rubber bands.   Elastic materials, for example, tension bands and surgical tubing, used to provide a source of external resistance for stretching and strengthening muscles.

sagittal plane.   The plane that runs from the front to the back of the body.

Actions such as flexion, extension, and hyperextension occur in the sagittal plane.

scapular downward rotation. Rotation of the scapula so that the lower point of the scapula moves toward the spine or midline of the body.

Shiatsu practitioner. One who uses the method of Shiatsu, or pressure points, in a therapeutic setting.

shinsplints. A stress condition of the lower leg that results in pain, swelling, and soreness of the muscles.

sickling. Pointing the foot—or plantar flexion—without equal tension on both sides of the ankle; the foot appears to be inverted (i.e., as if more weight is placed on its outer edge).

spinal discs. Cartilaginous discs that lie between the vertebrae to provide cushioning and shock absorption.

sprain. Injury to soft and connective tissues surrounding a joint, resulting in stretching or tearing of the ligaments with ensuing pain, swelling, and sometimes bruising.

static flexibility. The passive range of motion possible at a joint or series of joints.

strain. Injury to muscle resulting in pain, swelling, and bruising.

strapping, taping. Using tape or other materials to provide external support during the healing process.

stress fracture. Fracture (break) of a bone caused by repeated stress or overuse. Stress fractures are accompanied by pain and inflammation of the surrounding tissue, and may be difficult to diagnose.

supination. Of the foot: lifting the inside edge of the foot; also called rolling out (*q.v.*) or sickling (*q.v.*). Of the forearm: outward rotation of the lower arm that turns the palm away from the body.

supine. Lying face up.

surgical tubing. Elastic tubing used to provide resistance for strengthening.

talocalcaneal or **subtalar joint.** The joint between the talus (the ankle bone) and the calcaneus (the heel).

talus. The ankle bone. The talus articulates with the tibia and fibula to create the ankle joint.

taping. See **strapping.**

tendinitis. Inflammation of the tendon, resulting in pain, restricted motion, and crepitus within the tendon sheath.

teres major. A thick muscle that originates on the lower portion of the scapula, runs under the armpit, and attaches to the front of the humerus.

torque (moment of force). In common usage, torque refers to a rotary or twisting force. Technically, a torque (of a lever) is the product of the force and the moment arm.

torsion. The amount of twist inherent in a structure, such as a bone or a joint. Femoral torsion, the amount of twist inherent in the thigh bone, affects the amount of natural rotation (internal and external) of the leg. Less than 12 degrees of femoral torsion is called retroversion (*q.v.*); greater than 12 degrees of torsion is called anteversion (see **angle of femoral anteversion**). Tibial torsion is the amount of external twist intrinsic to the tibia. Excessive tibial torsion can create knee problems. Tibial torsion less than 12 degrees contributes to pigeontoed gait and pronation (*q.v.*).

traction. A pulling force.

transverse or **horizontal plane.** The plane that runs parallel to the ground. Actions such as internal and external rotation occur in the transverse plane.

ultrasound. A therapeutic device that employs high-frequency sound waves.

valgus (common usage). In the knees: knees are pointed inward, giving a knock-kneed appearance. In the foot: foot has a rolled-in appearance.

varus (common usage). In the knees: knees are apart, giving a bowlegged appearance. In the foot: foot looks as if it has a high arch.

winging. Eversion of the foot, accompanied by plantar flexion. Commonly employed to give the desired line to the leg in arabesque.

Notes

Preface

1. Interview on ABC *News*, "Person of the Week" segment, May 11, 1990.

Chapter 1

1. Gigi Berardi, "The Redesigning of a Dancer's Body," *Los Angeles Times*, 18 March 1990: 60. According to Bruce Marks, artistic director of the Boston Ballet, "We're getting away from that lithe, elongated look in ballet. . . . So not only do dancers have to dance differently, they have to look different."

2. Dr. Bert Mandelbaum, personal interview, May 3, 1989. Dr. Mandelbaum, who is assistant professor of orthopedic surgery at University of California, Los Angeles, attends to many of the athletes and dancers at UCLA. He is especially concerned for the dancers, noting that "Dancers would do anything to keep performing."

3. Dancers aren't simply "victims" of medical professionals. Anti-inflammatory, over-the-counter drugs enable dancers to keep moving. Ibuprofen, marketed under various trademark names, has probably done as much for dance as sprung wood flooring, making it possible to leap and jump and somersault even when injured. According to David Howard, international ballet master and coach, it's not unusual for dancers to live on ibuprofen, taking four or five

tablets in one dose. This is very disconcerting, given the volume of literature reporting harmful effects of the drug, in particular, potential renal toxicity. Dancers cannot take ibuprofen without jeopardizing their health.

4. David Howard recalls working on Baryshnikov's foot for forty-five minutes before one performance of *Coppélia*. Despite advice to the contrary, the dancer insisted on taping the irritated and inflamed foot and going on with the performance.

5. Of course, there are many other stressors besides injury in the dancer's life—domestic pressures, the death of colleagues and mentors, and even natural disasters. On October 17, 1989, San Francisco suffered a major earthquake. The San Francisco Ballet was performing in southern California as scheduled, not knowing if they had homes or family to return to.

6. Oleg Briansky, personal interview, May 6, 1989. Eight performances per week would not be uncommon for the Big Two (NYCB and American Ballet Theatre), the Big Three or Four (add The Joffrey Ballet and a favorite major regional company of choice), or for Broadway shows. Smaller audiences for modern dance companies generally mean smaller payrolls, smaller company size, and fewer performances, although it's difficult to generalize.

7. Merrill Ashley, telephone interview, September 5, 1987. Subsequent quotes of Merrill Ashley are taken from her book, *Dancing for Balanchine* (New York: E.P. Dutton, 1984), pp. 217–218.

8. Just four months after the Los Angeles performances, Ashley Wheater, Jerel Hilding, Glenn Edgerton, Leslie Carothers, and Patrick Corbin were no longer dancing with The Joffrey Ballet. These featured dancers left behind some big shoes to fill, which at the time added to performance pressures on the remaining soloists.

9. A case in point was that in 1989, negotiations to bring ABT to Los Angeles's Dorothy Chandler Pavilion for two weeks in July, nine years after its last engagement there, collapsed. According to ABT's executive director, Jane Hermann, "For a company of our size to go [to Los Angeles] unassisted by anyone—to be completely at risk, and yet have no ability to build a subscription audience was unacceptable [there was controversy about whether or not they would be allowed to perform for at least two consecutive years]." (Lewis Segal, "ABT cancels L.A. dates; frozen out by Joffrey?" *Los Angeles Times,* 20 December 1989: F-1, F-14.)

10. Differences in the total solids content of municipal drinking water can account for a large part of gastrointestinal illnesses that dancers

suffer. Water with a high solids load (over 500 mg/liter) can cause diarrhea or can sometimes have the opposite effect.

11. For example, Kenneth Laws, a professor of physics at Dickinson College in Carlisle, Pennsylvania, and author of *The physics of dance*, performs with the Central Pennsylvania Youth Ballet. He dances *The Nutcracker* each year and cameo roles at other times, or he may partner an up-and-coming ballerina in a spring performance. Laws in his mid-fifties continues to dance and perform.

12. I am using the term "professional" to describe individuals who earn their living in an occupation that is also engaged in by amateurs. The professional dancer should be performing on a somewhat regular basis in a Broadway show, film/video, school workshops, college auditoriums, a regional or nationally known ballet or modern dance company, and so forth. Using this definition, dancers who are full-time academic faculty would not be considered professional dancers, even though they may be performing three or four times a year. Strictly speaking, their salary is earned for teaching, service to the institution, and creative work, rather than for performance. Dancers who appear with small, less well-known companies, while earning their living elsewhere, might be termed "semiprofessional."

13. When bending the knees in a plié, it is the lengthening contraction of the knee extensors that allows the knee to bend smoothly. Strong quadriceps help to stabilize the knee joint and control the movement.

14. This practice dates from the 1860s. Before this time, pointe shoes were "unblocked," meaning that dancers padded their toes with cotton wool and stitched the tips of the shoes to provide added stability. Today, certain Soviet male dancers of Georgia and the Ukraine dance on pointe, with soft boots; the toes are unblocked. They actually dance with their toes flexed, thus landing directly on the ends of the metatarsals of the foot.

15. The lesser friction of pointe shoes allows the dancer to keep turning longer and with less difficulty. Pierina Legnani's celebrated thirty-two fouettés in *Aladdin*, *Cinderella*, and *Swan Lake* would have been even more difficult with the soft ballet slipper.

16. Larry Kaplan, "A conversation with Merrill Ashley," *Ballet Review* 17/1 (Spring 1989): 79–90.

17. Jay Seals, "Dance surfaces," in Allan J. Ryan and Robert E. Stephens, eds. *Dance medicine: A comprehensive guide*, Chapter 19 (Chicago: Pluribus Press, Inc./Minneapolis: The Physician and Sportsmedicine, 1987), p. 321.

18. Kenneth Laws, personal interview, July 25, 1989. See also Kenneth

Laws, "Physics and the potential for dance injury," *Medical Problems of Performing Artists* 1/3 (1986): 88.

19. At the very least, pushing the body image to its limits through use of laxatives and diuretics or by semistarvation is often counterproductive to maintaining low body fat (see Chapter 6).

20. This and the following quote are from pages 142 and 143 of Suzanne Gordon's highly readable and recommended *Off balance: The real world of ballet* (New York: Pantheon Books, 1983). The reader should note that it doesn't take an eating disorder to predispose a dancer to injury. Poor eating habits in general—dieting, low carbohydrate intake—can lead to fatigue and possible injury.

21. This and subsequent quotes are from pages 9 and 158 through 169 of L.M. Vincent's *Competing with the sylph: The quest for the perfect dance body,* 2nd ed. (Princeton, N.J.: Princeton Book Company, Publishers, 1989). This book is essential reading for anyone interested in a career in professional ballet and especially for any woman who has struggled to achieve that "perfect body."

22. Vincent actually refers to immature hormonal patterns induced by low body fat and strenuous exercise. Does this characterize the "perfect" Balanchine ballerina? Probably. According to Gelsey Kirkland and Greg Lawrence, "Mr. B's ideal proportions called for an almost skeletal frame, accentuating the collarbones and length of the neck. Defeminization was the overall result, with the frequent cessation of the menstrual cycle due to malnutrition and physical abuse" (*Dancing on my grave* [Garden City, N.Y.: Doubleday, 1986], p. 56). For a scholarly review of this subject, see L.M. Vincent, "Body and mind: Adaptations and natural selection in ballet," *Kinesiology and Medicine for Dance* 13/1 (1990–1991): 33-46.

23. According to Dr. Eivind Thomasen of Sweden, this is not necessarily the case in Europe, where dancers retire in their forties and fifties.

24. Throughout their lives, dancers stretch and condition their bodies to achieve a desired line—perfect turnout or beautiful hip hyperextension. While they dance, their muscles are strong to stabilize the hip joint. However, when they stop dancing and become physically inactive, the muscles weaken. The ligaments are no longer functioning to stabilize the hip joint. This in turn causes instability of the joint and accentuates the arthritic wear-and-tear process.

25. Within six months, the second of Balanchine's personally groomed ballerinas to retire was Suzanne Farrell, at age forty-four.

26. Francis Mason, "Celebrating Patricia McBride," *Ballet Review* 17/1 (Spring 1989): 35.

27. Daniel Nagrin, *How to dance forever: Surviving against the odds* (New York: William Morrow, 1988), pp. 359, 18.

28. Ibid., p. 17.

29. Ibid., p. 21.

30. Ibid., p. 28.

31. Ibid., pp. 37, 40.

32. Jack Turner, "Art and injury: ABT's Raymond Serrano talks about the agony of ballet," *Massage Therapy Journal,* Fall 1988: 20–23.

33. Nagrin, p. 41.

34. Ibid., p. 44.

Chapter 2

1. The relationship to career longevity is clear. Robert Stephens points out that "very few dancers escape the tragedy of careers cut short by injury. . . . The dancer's 'Achilles heel' is a reluctance to face the need for effective injury prevention programs. . . . To do so would admit to one's own vulnerabilities—a disturbing thought when one is preoccupied with the ferocious demands of acquiring and maintaining . . . technique" (*Dance medicine: A comprehensive guide* [Chicago: Pluribus Press/Minneapolis: The Physician and Sportsmedicine, 1987], p. 16).

2. See L.M. Vincent, *The dancer's book of health* (Princeton, N.J.: Princeton Book Company, Publishers, 1978), Chapter 4, for a complete discussion.

3. For an excellent discussion of rehabilitative upper body exercise, see *Medicine and Science in Sports and Exercise: Special Symposium Issue,* 21/5 (1989): S119–S157.

4. For in-depth discussions of psoas insufficiency syndrome and lower-back dysfunction, see works by R.M. Bachrach, M. Molnar, and A.J. Ryan and R.E. Stephens in the Bibliography. Also, related strengthening and flexibility exercises are illustrated in Chapter 4. It is essential that the deeper abdominal muscles, the internal and external obliques, and the transversus abdominis be strengthened in any abdominal conditioning program (see J. Gantz, "The relationship between intra-abdominal pressure and dance training," *Kinesiology for Dance* 9/4 [1987]: 15–18).

5. Nerve palsy can result from extended treatment of two hours or more. G. Green and colleagues have reported on palsy resulting from shorter time intervals ("Peroneal nerve palsy induced by cryotherapy," *The Physician and Sportsmedicine* 17/9 [1989]: 63–70). In their

case study, the extent to which damage was caused by the cold temperature after application of the ice pack is unclear; compression of nerves by the elastic bandages was perhaps to blame. As long as the injured area is checked five to ten minutes after application (and regularly thereafter) of the wrap, there should be little cause for concern.

6. Daniel Nagrin, *How to dance forever: Surviving against the odds* (New York: William Morrow and Company, Inc., 1988), p. 175.

7. See ibid., pp. 119–166 for commentary on the healing options. Few of the treatments are inexpensive; many are not covered by insurance.

8. All statements by Raymond Serrano are from Jack Turner, "Art and injury: The ABT's Raymond Serrano talks about the agony of ballet," *Massage Therapy Journal*, Fall 1988: 22.

9. Irmgard Bartenieff, with Dori Lewis, *Body movement: Coping with the environment* (New York: Gordon and Breach Science Publishers, 1980), pp. 229–259.

10. Martha Myers and Marian Horosko, "When classes are not enough: Body Therapies—why, which, and when," *Dance Magazine*, July 1989: 47.

11. Training in Bartenieff Fundamentals is available through the Laban/Bartenieff Institute for Movement Studies (New York, Seattle) and "extension" programs in other cities (e.g., Los Angeles).

12. Lulu E. Sweigard, *Human movement potential: Its ideokinetic facilitation* (New York: Harper & Row, Publishers, 1974).

13. Sweigard, p. 233.

14. Ibid., p. 237.

15. Ibid., pp. 238–239.

16. Ibid., p. 239.

17. Irene Dowd certifies teachers of ideokinesis at her studio in New York.

18. F. Matthias Alexander, *The universal constant in living* (New York: Dutton, 1941), p. 10.

19. Accredited training programs are approved by organizations such as the North American Society of Teachers of the Alexander Technique (NASTAT), the American Center for the Alexander Technique (ACAT), and the Society of Teachers of the Alexander Technique (STAT) in London.

20. Eleanor Rosenthal, "The Alexander technique—What it is and how it works," *Medical Problems of Performing Artists*, June 1987: 55.

Rosenthal is a past president and director of the American Center for the Alexander Technique.

21. Martha Myers, "Body therapies and the modern dancer: The Alexander technique," *Dance Magazine,* April 1980: 92.

22. Martha Myers, personal communication, February 20, 1990.

23. Moshe Feldenkrais, *Awareness through movement* (New York: Harper & Row, Publishers, 1972).

24. Ibid., pp. 80–82.

25. One can train in Feldenkrais method with certified practitioners or by using *Awareness through movement.*

26. Judy Gantz, "Evaluation of faulty dance technique patterns: A working model," *Kinesiology and Medicine for Dance* 12/1 (1989): 1–11.

27. Alan J. Ryan and Robert E. Stephens, *The dancer's complete guide to healthcare and a long career* (Chicago: Bonus Books, 1988), pp. 162–163.

28. For a complete discussion of tendinitis around the ankle joint (Richard Braver refers to it as tendinitis *rond de ankle* since the inflammation may involve many tendons), see the five-part series published in *Kinesiology for Dance* 10/4–11/4 (1988–89).

29. See also Terry R. Malone and William Hardaker, "Rehabilitation of foot and ankle injuries in ballet dancers," *Journal of Orthopaedic and Sports Physical Therapy* 11/8 (1990): 355–361.

30. For an extensive discussion of impingement syndrome and its treatment, see L.A. Thein, "Impingement syndrome and its conservative management," *The Journal of Orthopaedic and Sports Physical Therapy* 11/5 (1989): 183–191.

31. For a review of the literature on specific exercises, see ibid., pp. 189–190.

32. For a comprehensive discussion of the syndrome and its treatment at NYCB, see Elizabeth Henry, "Treatment of posterior compression of the lower lumbar spine in male ballet dancers," *Kinesiology and Medicine for Dance* 12/2 (1989): 22–31.

33. Daniel Nagrin gives a detailed account of his preperformance ritual as an aid to younger performers in developing their own (*How to dance forever,* pp. 38–41).

34. For a good discussion of warm-up objectives and characteristics, see D.B. Franks, "Physical warm-up," in W.P. Morgan, ed. *Ergogenic aids and muscular performance* (New York: Academic Press, 1972), pp. 159–191; A. Grodjinovsky and J.R. Magel, "Effect of warm-up

on running performance," *Research Quarterly* 41/1 (1970): 116–117.

35. See Debbie and Carlos Rosas, with Katherine Martin, *Nonimpact aerobics* (New York: Avon Books, 1987).

36. Merrill Ashley, *Dancing for Balanchine* (New York: E.P. Dutton, Inc., 1984). All subsequent quotes are taken from this source.

37. Ibid., pp. 217–218.

Chapter 3

1. Stuart Wright, *Dancer's guide to injuries of the lower extremity* (New York: Cornwall Books, 1985), p. 14.

2. Ruth Solomon and Lyle Micheli, "Concepts in the prevention of dance injuries: A survey and analysis," in Caroline G. Shell, ed. *The dancer as athlete,* Chapter 21 (Champaign, Ill.: Human Kinetics, 1986); Karen Clippinger-Robertson, Robert Hutton, Doris Miller, and T. Richard Nichols, "Mechanical and anatomical factors relating to the incidence and etiology of patellofemoral pain in dancers," ibid., Chapter 5.

3. See Judy Gantz, "The relationship between intra-abdominal pressure and dance training," *Kinesiology for Dance* 9/4 (1987): 15–18.

4. Kenneth Laws, *The physics of dance* (New York: Schirmer Books, 1984), p. 9.

5. For an excellent discussion of biomechanics applied to dance, see Priscilla M. Clarkson and Margaret Skrinar, eds. *Science of dance training,* Chapter 8 (Champaign, Ill.: Human Kinetics, 1988). For further discussion of dance kinesiology, see the following articles in *Kinesiology for Dance:* Kenneth Laws, "Dance kinesiology—difficulties and directions" (No. 1 [October 1984]: 6–7); Sue Stigleman, "Dance kinesiology: The field and its literature" (No. 15 [June 1981]: 5–9); and Sally Fitt, "The Importance of Kinesiology for Dancers" (No. 1 [May 1977]: 6–7). *Kinesiology for Dance* is a journal devoted entirely to the study of dance science in human movement. Since 1977, it has published articles ranging from the art of centering to the effect of plyometric training on dancers' vertical jump height to medical treatment for common skin lesions of the feet. Now as a refereed journal and with an expanded title, *Kinesiology and Medicine for Dance,* the journal is published by Princeton Periodicals, Inc., in Pennington, New Jersey.

6. See Lyle J. Micheli and Ruth Solomon, "Training the young dancer," in Allan J. Ryan and Robert E. Stephens, eds. *Dance medicine: A*

comprehensive guide, Chapter 3 (Chicago: Pluribus Press, Inc./ Minneapolis: The Physician and Sportsmedicine, 1987), p. 60.

7. Dancers often speak of "torques" on the body. Daniel Nagrin gives a good definition of torque as it is sometimes used in dance (*How to dance forever: Surviving against the odds* [New York: William Morrow and Company, Inc., 1988], p. 96). He describes a torque at the knee—on one part of the body from another—which could possibly injure the knee.

8. For further discussion, see Lei Li, with Kenneth Laws, "The physical analysis of *Da She Yan Tiao,*" *Kinesiology for Dance* 11/4 (1989): 9–11; Kenneth Laws and Kyong Lee, "The *grand jeté:* A physical analysis," ibid., pp. 12–13.

9. Kenneth Laws, "Physics and the potential for dance injury," *Medical Problems of Performing Artists* 1/3 (1986): 88.

10. See the excellent discussion by Kenneth Laws regarding the timing of the extension of the arms and legs. Laws explains how, when the arms are almost straight, a greater vertical force may be exerted (*The physics of dance,* pp. 99–100).

11. For an excellent discussion of the knee, see Ronald Quirk, "The dancer's knee," in Allan J. Ryan and Robert E. Stephens, eds. *Dance medicine: A comprehensive guide,* Chapter 11 (Chicago: Pluribus Press, Inc./Minneapolis: The Physician and Sportsmedicine, 1987); for femoral angle and torsion, tibial torsion, and limited plantarflexion due to different anatomical variations, see Robert E. Stephens, "The etiology of injuries in ballet," ibid., Chapter 2.

12. Karen Clippinger-Robertson, "Flexibility in dance," *Kinesiology and Medicine for Dance* 12/2 (1990): 1–16, and *Flexibility for aerobics and fitness* (Seattle, Wash.: Seattle Sports Medicine, 1987).

13. Judy Gantz, "Evaluation of faulty dance technique patterns: A working model," *Kinesiology and Medicine for Dance* 12/1 (1989): 1–11. Gantz goes on to discuss how to define and identify faulty dance coordination patterns and develop a working framework of analysis to assess faulty technique.

14. For further discussion on choosing technique teachers, see Margaret Skrinar, "Who's teaching the technique class?" in Priscilla M. Clarkson and Margaret Skrinar, eds. *Science of dance training,* Chapter 16 (Champaign, Ill.: Human Kinetics Publishers, Inc., 1988); Micheli and Solomon.

15. Joseph Mazo, "Erick Hawkins: Still tapping the sap of spring," *New York Times,* 26 November 1989, Section 2: 12, 32.

16. Laws, *The physics of dance,* p. xii.

Chapter 4

1. Karen Clippinger-Robertson, "Principles of dance training," in Priscilla M. Clarkson and Margaret Skrinar, eds. *Science of dance training* (Champaign, Ill.: Human Kinetics Publishers, Inc., 1988), p. 45.

2. See Gigi Berardi, "The redesigning of a dancer's body," *Los Angeles Times,* 18 March 1990: 60, 62.

3. Also see Katherine C. Buroker and James A. Schwane, "Does postexercise static stretching alleviate delayed muscle soreness?" *The Physician and Sportsmedicine* 17/6 (1989): 65–83.

4. See Niels Bukh, Emily R. Andrews, and Karen Vesterdal, *Fundamental gymnastics: The basis of rational physical development* (New York: E.P. Dutton & Co., 1928), pp. ix–x, 2.

5. It is interesting to see how much of Hawkins's work is a logical progression from the Bukh gymnastics work: Bukh et al. write about "continuous work proceeding from one exercise to another without stopping [in which] unison need not be stressed . . . extension without tension" (*Fundamental gymnastics*, pp. 2, 15).

6. Kathryn Karipides, personal interview, Case Western Reserve University, June 25, 1988.

7. See R.M. Bachrach, "Injuries to the dancer's spine," in Allan J. Ryan and Robert E. Stephens, eds. *Dance medicine: A comprehensive guide,* Chapter 13 (Chicago: Pluribus Press, Inc./Minneapolis: The Physician and Sportsmedicine, 1987).

8. For a history of GAS dating back to 1936, see Hans Selye, *The stress of life* (New York: McGraw-Hill, 1976); see also his *Stress without distress* (New York: J.P. Lippincott, 1974).

9. See John Garhammer, *Sports Illustrated strength training* (New York: Harper & Row, Publishers, 1986), pp. 152–153.

10. Clippinger-Robertson, "Principles of dance training," p. 50.

11. For further discussion, see Clippinger-Robertson, "Principles of dance training," pp. 51, 64; Garhammer, pp. 29–32.

12. Also to enhance flexibility, the muscles should be worked throughout their full range of motion. This is relatively easy to do with free weights.

13. For more information, see Garhammer, pp. 189–199; and Donald Chu, "Planned progression," *Idea Today* 7/8 (September 1989): 30–35.

14. For additional information and guidelines when using the bands, see Patricia A. VanGalen, *Exercising with DYNA-BAND total body*

toner: Basic guidelines for the instructor (Akron, Ohio: The Hygienic Corporation, 1987). Note that all exercises should be performed only after a suitable warm-up.

15. Gantz suggests up to fifteen reps for as many as four or five days a week. This frequency may be a little high, depending on the resistance that is used. For a discussion, see Garhammer, Chapters 5 and 7.

16. See M.H. Stone and H. Bryant, *Weight training, a scientific approach* (Minneapolis: Burgess International Group, Inc., 1987).

17. This is an example, rather than a blanket endorsement, of Cybex equipment used for strengthening regimens.

18. Studies by Kent Timm ("Postsurgical knee rehabilitation: A five-year study of four methods and 5,381 patients," *American Journal of Sports Medicine* 16/5 [1988]: 463–468) and Michael J. Smith and Paul Melton ("Isokinetic versus isotonic variable-resistance training," ibid., 9/4 [1981]: 275–279) have shown that isokinetic training—the resistance mechanism of the Cybex machines in which a constant speed of motion is maintained—is especially useful in rehabilitation to restore motor performance skills such as running and jumping.

    In a general conditioning program there are other considerations. Exercising at a constant movement speed (as opposed to exercising with acceleration as with free weights) means that no acceleration is present, and in this sense it is not specific to real-life dance movement patterns. However, the advantages offered by the machines—convenience, safety control, training at high speeds—outweigh the disadvantages, especially if strength-training programs use a combination of free weights and machines. For further discussion, see Garhammer, pp. 53 ff.

19. For further discussion, see Robin D. Chmelar, Sally S. Fitt, and Susan S. Smith, "Isokinetic characteristics of the knee and trunk in ballet and modern dancers," paper presented at the Seventh Annual Symposium on Medical Problems of Musicians and Dancers, Snowmass, Colorado, August 3–6, 1989.

20. The cam varies the distance from its axle pivot to the point where force is being applied.

21. For an excellent discussion, see Maria Junco, "Pilates technique," *Dance Teacher Now* 10/9 (1988): 27–30.

22. The material discussed in this section is taken principally from Garhammer, pp. 114–129.

23. This lift is usually performed with a barbell. For further instructions and for cautionary notes, see Garhammer, pp. 127–129.

24. Bruce Marks, telephone interview, January 30, 1989.

25. See J.L. Cohen, P.K. Gupta, E. Lichistein, and K.D. Chadda, "The heart of a dancer: Noninvasive cardiac evaluation of professional ballet dancers," *American Journal of Cardiology* 45 (1980): 959–965. See also Bibliography.

26. To obtain an estimate of maximal heart rate (also called "maximum exercise heart rate"), subtract the person's age from 220 (e.g., the maximal attainable heart rate of a thirty-year-old is 220 − 30 or about 190). For a more accurate estimate of calculating maximal and training heart rates, see Sally Fitt, *Dance kinesiology* (New York: Schirmer Books, 1988), Chapters 14, 19. Note that the heart rate can actually go higher than 80 percent; some highly trained athletes work at levels higher than "220 minus their age," but it is not safe to do so for many individuals. Exercise at 70 percent is often referred to as "conversational exercise" (i.e., it is possible to hold a conversation while exercising without being exhausted).

27. J.L. Cohen, K.R. Segal, I. Witriol, and W.D. McArdle, "Cardiorespiratory responses to ballet exercise and the VO_2max of elite ballet dancers," *Medicine and Science in Sports and Exercise* 14 (1982): 212–217.

28. This point is highly disputed among dance kinesiologists and exercise physiologists. The physiologists argue that one hour of intense interval-burst anaerobic activity will, over a twenty-four-hour life period, "burn" more fat than one hour of aerobic endurance training over the same twenty-four-hour life period. The former exercise simply mobilizes more fat after the workout (this can be hours later), the latter *during* the workout. Few people, however, can sustain an intense interval-burst anaerobic activity for even one hour.

29. See Steven Chatfield and William C. Byrnes, "Cardiovascular aspects of dance," in Priscilla M. Clarkson and Margaret Skrinar, eds. *Science of dance training,* Chapter 6 (Champaign, Ill.: Human Kinetics Publishers, Inc., 1988).

30. Ibid., pp. 103–104.

31. See Debbie C. Lieber, Richard L. Lieber, and William C. Adams, "Effects of run-training and swim-training at similar absolute intensities on treadmill VO_2max," *Medicine and Science in Sports and Exercise* 21/6 (1989): 655–661. Whether or not there is "transfer" in aerobic capacity from cycling to running to swim training is controversial.

32. Dennis M. Davidson, "Dance and cardiorespiratory fitness," in Caroline G. Shell, ed. *The dancer as athlete: The 1984 Olympic scientific congress proceedings* (Champaign, Ill.: Human Kinetics

Publishers, Inc., 1986), p. 137. Swimming is excellent exercise as long as the dancer's speed and quickness needed in performance is not affected (see Daniel Nagrin, *How to dance forever*, p. 138). Also, to avoid shoulder and back problems, dancers should be certain that their upper body is properly conditioned before embarking on a swimming regimen.

33. This increase was approximately eight percent. These data were for a nondance population. See the short review article by Bryant Stamford, "How much should I exercise?" *The Physician and Sportsmedicine* 17/7 (1989): 150.

34. The results are conflicting as to whether or not intermittent versus continuous exercise results in greater caloric expenditure over a twenty-four-hour life period. The reason the intermittent may be more effective is that the participant gets tired and works less hard with continuous and heavy exercise.

35. Steven N. Blair, Harold W. Kohl III, Ralph S. Paffenbarger, Debra G. Clark, Kenneth H. Cooper, and Larry W. Gibbons, "Physical fitness and all-cause mortality: A prospective study of healthy men and women," *Journal of the American Medical Association* 262/17 (1989): 2395–2401.

36. Weak inward rotators may be secondary to structural problems in causing injury, for example retroversion of the neck of the femur, resulting in the "toed-out" running.

37. For further information, see Debbie Rosas and Carlos Rosas, with Katherine Martin, *Nonimpact aerobics* (New York: Avon Books, 1988).

38. For further discussion, see J.P. Clausen, "Effect of physical training on cardiovascular adjustments to exercise in men," *Physiological Reviews* 57 (1977): 779.

39. For more information, see Robin Chmelar and Sally Fitt, *Dancing at your peak: Diet* (Princeton, N.J.: Princeton Book Co., Publishers, 1990).

40. See Clippinger-Robertson, "Principles of dance training," p. 60.

41. See Karen Clippinger-Robertson, "Flexibility in dance," *Kinesiology and Medicine for Dance* 12/2 (1990): 1.

42. See T. Hortobagyi, J. Faludi, J. Tohanyi, and B. Merkeley, "Effects of intense 'stretching'-flexibility training on the mechanical profile of the knee extensors and on the range of motion of the hip joint," *Int. Journal Sports Med.* 6 (1985): 317–321.

43. For a very interesting discussion of the neurophysiology of flexibility,

see Michael Alter, *Science of stretching*, Chapter 5 (Champaign, Ill.: Human Kinetics Publishers, Inc., 1988), pp. 43–50; and Robert Stephens, "The neuroanatomical and biomechanical basis of flexibility exercises in dance," in R. Solomon, S. Minton, and J. Solomon, eds. *Preventing dance injuries: An interdisciplinary perspective*, Chapter 13 (Reston, Va.: American Alliance for Health, Physical Education, Recreation and Dance, 1990), pp. 271–92.

44. See Robert Stephens's excellent discussion of the difference between elastic deformation of tissue, occurring within the muscle cell, and the longer-lasting plastic deformation, occurring in the connective tissue (ibid., pp. 284–285).

45. See G.H. Van Gyn, "Contemporary stretching techniques: Theory and application," in Caroline G. Shell, ed. *The dancer as athlete: The 1984 Olympic scientific congress proceedings*, Chapter 10 (Champaign, Ill: Human Kinetics Publishers, Inc., 1986).

46. See N. Wolkodoff, "Physiology and application of flexibility programs," paper presented at the IDEA One-to-One Fitness Conference, Los Angeles, California, April 14–16, 1989.

47. H. Kabat first developed the methods in his clinical work; L.E. Holt and colleagues applied them to general conditioning regimens. (See Bibliography.)

48. There is some debate over exactly how long this stretch should be held—perhaps not more than five seconds—to reduce the risk of delayed muscle soreness.

49. For further discussion, see Van Gyn.

50. See Michael Alter, Chapter 11, for a more complete discussion of the pros and cons of passive and active stretching.

51. Judy Alter, *Stretch and strengthen* (Boston: Houghton Mifflin, 1986) and *Surviving exercise: Judy Alter's safe and sane exercise program* (Boston: Houghton Mifflin, 1983).

52. Adapted from Ruth Lindsey and Charles Corbin, "Questionable exercises—some safer alternatives," *Journal of Physical Education, Recreation and Dance* 60/8 (1989): 26–32.

53. Adapted from Judy Alter. See also Karen Clippinger-Robertson, "Components of an aerobic dance-exercise class," in *Aerobic dance-exercise instructor manual* (San Diego: IDEA Foundation, 1987), Chapter 5; Elizabeth Stevenson, "Hyperflexion of the knee," *CAHPERD Journal Times* 52/2 (1989): 21–22. Lindsey and Corbin also offer an excellent discussion of other exercises to avoid, such as double leg lifts, donkey kicks, and deep squatting exercises.

54. A very interesting dialogue regarding "potentially dangerous" exercises has been conducted by Karen Clippinger-Robertson, one of dance science's foremost proponents, and physician-editor James Garrick, among others. An important point emerges from this debate: if work with professional athletes and dancers is one-on-one in a clinical setting, some potentially dangerous exercises are not that "dangerous" (see Lubell in Bibliography).

55. See Michael Alter, p. 115, for a discussion of further modifications of the hurdler's stretch.

56. See Allan J. Ryan and Robert E. Stephens, *The dancer's complete guide to healthcare and a long career* (Chicago: Bonus Books, 1988), pp. 169–196.

57. Some typical exercises modified to accommodate the less flexible dancer are (1) Deep Calf Stretch: from a seated position, the right knee is bent and the right foot is actively held and flexed (I would add that to increase the stretch, the lower spine should fully press into the thigh and the right foot should be maximally flexed; hold the ball of the foot rather than the toes; repeat with the left leg and foot), and (2) Standing Deep Hip Flexor Stretch at the Barre: the body leans (tombé) toward the barre, with the torso nearly vertical; the pelvis is pressed toward the barre. (For illustrations, see ibid., pp. 185–196).

58. Karen Clippinger-Robertson, *Flexibility for aerobics and fitness* (Seattle: Seattle Sports Medicine, 1987).

59. Clippinger-Robertson, "Flexibility in dance," pp. 1–16.

60. Kelly Holt, *Graduate dance training program bulletin* (Cleveland: Case Western Reserve University, Department of Theatre, Drama and Dance, 1984).

Chapter 5

1. Some researchers estimate the percentage of calories from fat in dancers' diets to be as high as two-thirds; the average for the United States population is closer to 40 percent. See Jane M. Bonbright, "The nutritional status of female ballet dancers 15–18 years of age," *Dance Research Journal* 21/2 (1989): 9–14. See also Bibliography (Benson et al. [1985], Bright-See et al., Calabrese et al., Cohen et al.).

2. L.M. Vincent, "Dancers and the war with water and salt," *Kinesiology and Medicine for Dance* 12/2 (1990): 40–49, and *Competing with the sylph*, 2nd ed. (Princeton, N.J.: Princeton Book Company, Publishers, 1989). See also Sharon A. Armann, Christine L. Wells, Susanne S. Cheung, Stuart L. Posner, Ronald J. Fischer,

Judith A. Pachtman, and Russell P. Chick, "Bone mass, menstrual abnormalities, dietary intake, and body composition in classical ballerinas," *Kinesiology and Medicine for Dance* 13/1 (1990): 1–15.

3. Bonbright, pp. 12–13.

4. Ibid., pp. 11–12.

5. For an excellent discussion of energy nutrients and energy metabolism, see Frank I. Katch and William D. McArdle, *Nutrition, weight control, and exercise* (Philadelphia: Lea & Febiger, 1988), Chapters 1 and 4.

6. See Paul McCarthy, "How much protein do athletes really need?" *The Physician and Sportsmedicine* 17/5 (1989): 170–175; J.R. Brotherhood, "Nutrition and sports performance," *Sports Med.*, Sept.–Oct. 1984: 350–389; L.H. Hamilton, J. Brooks-Gunn, and M.P. Warren, "Nutritional intake of female dancers: A reflection of eating problems," *International Journal of Eating Disorders* 5 (1986): 925–934.

7. Joanne L. Slavin, Greg Lanners, and Mark A. Engstrom, "Amino acid supplements: Beneficial or risky?" *The Physician and Sportsmedicine* 16/3 (1988): 222.

8. AHA (American Heart Association), *Heart cuisine* (Los Angeles, Cal.: AHA, undated), pp. 121–122.

9. National Research Council, *Recommended dietary allowances,* 1980, pp. 166, 168. See also the general discussion in the tenth edition of the Council's *Recommended dietary allowances* and in its *Diet and health,* both published in 1989 by the National Academy of Sciences (National Academy Press).

10. See L.M. Vincent, "Dancers and the war with water and salt."

11. See Eric T. Poehlman, "A review: Exercise and its influence on resting energy metabolism in man," *Medicine and Science in Sports and Exercise* 21/5 (1989): 515–525.

12. For a review of the evidence supporting a significant genetic component affecting RMR (after accounting for the effects of age, gender, and body composition), see Poehlman.

13. See Katch and McArdle, pp. 102–103.

14. See Paul A. Mole, Judith S. Stern, Cynthia L. Schultz, Edmund M. Bernauer, and Bryan J. Holcomb, "Exercise reverses depressed metabolic rate produced by severe caloric restriction," *Medicine and Science in Sports and Exercise* 2/1 (1989): 29–33. The study showed that with thirty minutes of daily exercise at 60 percent VO_2max, energy expenditure can be stimulated. The trend in loss of lean body

mass can be reversed so that most of the weight lost (over 80 percent) is fat, not muscle. However, these data have more relevance for diseased subjects (obese individuals) than for athletes and dancers, who should not engage in severe caloric restriction, especially of carbohydrates.

15. National Research Council (NRC), *Recommended dietary allowances*, 1980, p. 1.

16. E.R. Pariser and M. Wallerstein, "Fish protein concentrate: Lessons for future food supplementation" (1980), in Gigi M. Berardi, ed. *World food, population and development*, Chapter 37 (Totowa, N.J.: Rowman and Allanheld, 1985), p. 243.

17. Michael Latham, "Nutrition and infection in national development" (1975), in ibid., Chapter 34, pp. 233–234.

18. National Research Council, ibid., p. 17.

19. AHA (American Heart Association), *Heart cuisine* (Los Angeles, Cal.: AHA, undated).

20. Ibid.

21. Robin Chmelar and Sally Fitt, *Dancing at your peak: Diet* (Princeton, N.J.: Princeton Book Co., Publishers, 1990). Note, however, that many female dancers have difficulty trying to lose weight with protein intakes below 15 percent of calories, when the total caloric intake is less than 1,200 kcal.

22. Bonbright, p. 12.

23. See Mole et al.

24. See J.B. Van Itallie and M. Yang, "Current concepts in nutrition: Diet and weight loss," *New England Journal of Medicine* 297 (1977): 1158–1161.

25. Bonbright, p. 11.

26. For a good discussion of body fat and dance, see Chmelar and Fitt.

27. For a comprehensive discussion of fuel homeostasis, see Harriet Wallberg-Henriksson, "Acute exercise: Fuel homeostasis and glucose transport in insulin-dependent diabetes mellitus," *Medicine and Science in Sports and Exercise* 21/4 (1989): 356–361.

28. See Darlene A. Sedlock, Jean A. Fissinger, and Christopher L. Melby, "Effect of exercise intensity and duration on postexercise energy expenditure," *Medicine and Science in Sports and Exercise* 21/6 (1989): 662–666. For a review of the literature on the extent to which purposeful physical exercise (by trained and untrained individuals) can increase basal or resting energy expenditure, see Poehlman, and Wallberg-Henriksson.

29. Katch and McArdle, p. 94.

30. For an excellent discussion of muscle structure and energy systems, see John Garhammer, *Sports Illustrated strength training* (New York: Harper & Row, 1986), pp. 29–32.

31. For a good discussion on this compulsive behavior, see "Overcoming the ten-pound obsession," *Tufts University Diet and Nutrition Letter* 6/11 (1989): 3–6.

32. Allegra Kent, with James and Constance Camner, *The dancers' body book* (New York: William Morrow and Company, Inc., 1984), p. 59.

33. Ibid.

34. See Chmelar and Fitt.

35. Dr. Steven Scheck, personal communication, February 27, 1990. Dr. Scheck is in the Department of Biology at Loyola Marymount University, Los Angeles, California.

36. Frances Munnings reports on a study with cyclists. The findings show that even though eating candy bars results in a drop of glucose levels below baseline levels, the time to exhaustion doesn't necessarily increase ("Candy before exercise: Not so bad after all?" *Physician and Sportsmedicine* 17/11 [1989]: 24, 26). Researchers conclude that the transient hypoglycemia doesn't impair performance, at least in high-intensity exercise. (Of course, it's not too surprising that this research was funded by the Hershey Foods Corp.) Still, it's better to choose orange juice before a high-fat candy bar.

Chapter 6

1. Dancers, however, share a strong internal locus of control over their training and their weight—so much so that their physical and emotional health is often in jeopardy. See Jerome M. Schnitt and Diana Schnitt, "Psychological issues in a dancer's career," in Allan J. Ryan and Robert E. Stephens, *Dance medicine: A comprehensive guide,* Chapter 20 (Chicago: Pluribus Press, Inc./Minneapolis: The Physician and Sportsmedicine, 1987).

2. Liz Lerman, *Fact sheet* (Washington, D.C.: Dance Exchange, undated), p. 1.

3. Tobi Tobias, [Liz Lerman review], *Washington Journal,* March 1988: 1.

4. Carol-Lynne Moore, "Body metaphors: Some implications for movement education," *Interchange* 18/3 (1987): 31–37.

5. Joanna Friesen, "Perceiving dance," *The Journal of Aesthetic Education* 9/4 (1975): 101.

6. Gloria Byron, "Making money talk—Part one: Who's got the goods?"; "Part two: How much is enough?" *Dance Magazine,* October–November 1989: 44–47; 40–43.

7. Byron (October 1989), p. 44.

8. Robert Sandla, "Money matters," *Dance Magazine,* March 1990: 74–75. Sandla's excellent article is particularly useful for New York–based choreographers and dance producers.

9. See Byron (November 1989), pp. 43, for a discussion of dancers' salaries compared with those of musicians, stagehands, and other artists and technicians. At issue is not just minimum salaries, but guaranteed work weeks—anywhere from thirty-eight to forty-four— as well as supplemental disability insurance, medical and dental insurance, and vacation pay. Dance companies operating under the National Basic Dance Agreement of the AFL-CIO–affiliated AGMA usually can guarantee dancers as many as forty weeks of work a year.

10. American Guild of Musical Artists, *AGMA Golden Jubilee* (New York: AGMA, 1986), p. 6.

11. American Guild of Musical Artists, pp. 9–10.

12. See Suzanne Gordon, *Off balance: The real world of ballet* (New York: McGraw Hill, 1983).

13. Since 1982, there have been at least three separate filings for arbitration with ABT. In one case, a ballerina (height 5'2"; weight 105 lbs.) had been "fired" because she was "fat." According to the labor lawyer, Leonard Leibowitz, this arbitration was easily won, since the firing was allegedly for "just cause," rather than "artistic reasons."

14. *New York Times,* 14 May 1990: p. B1.

15. See Gordon, page 190. Robin Chmelar—a research specialist for Cybex New York—has prepared "Data sheet on workers' compensation" for performing artists (New York: Center for Safety in the Arts, undated).

Bibliography

Dance: A Demanding Profession

Ashley, Merrill. *Dancing for Balanchine.* New York: E. P. Dutton, Inc., 1984.

Beier, W. "On a relationship between biological age and functional age," *Aktuel. Gerontol.* 11/3 (1981): 106–107.

Berardi, Gigi. "The agony of dancing," *Los Angeles Times,* 21 May 1989: 61–62.

Bortz, W. "Disuse and aging," *Journal of the American Medical Association* 248/10 (1982): 1203–1208.

Breslauer, Jan. "Dancer meditates on growing older in 'Ancient Terrain,' " *Los Angeles Times,* 24 June 1989: 4.

Cherebetiu, G., A. Islas, and J. Garcia. *Maximal anaerobic power in sedentary males between 20 and 65 years of age.* Mexico City, Mexico: National Center of Sport, Medicine and Applied Science, 1986.

De Vries, Herbert A. and Dianne Hales. *Fitness after 50: An exercise prescription for lifelong health.* New York: Charles Scribner's Sons, 1981.

Dolinar, Louis. "Ballet? MD finds it rough as any sport," *The Physician and Sports Medicine* November 1976: 87–92.

Drinkwater, B.L., S.M. Horvath, and C.L. Wells. "Aerobic power of females, ages 10 to 68," *J. Gerontol.* 30/4 (1975): 385–394.

Fitt, Sally S. *Dance kinesiology.* New York: Schirmer Books, 1988.

Fleg, J.L. "Alterations in cardiovascular structure and function with advancing age," *Am. J. Cardiol.* 57/5 (1986): 33C–44C.

Gomez, Ninoska. "Moving with somatic awareness: The body-mind centering approach to growth and health," *Journal of Physical Education, Recreation and Dance,* September 1988: 90–96.

Gordon, Suzanne. *Off balance: The real world of ballet.* New York: Pantheon Books, 1983.

Hagberg, J.M., W.K. Allen, and J.O. Holloszy. "A hemodynamic comparison of young and older endurance athletes during exercise," *J. Applied Physiology* 58/6 (1985): 2041–2046.

Hamilton, W.G. "Physical prerequisites for ballet dancers," *Musculoskeletal Medicine* 3 (1986): 61–66.

Hartley, A.A. and J.T. Hartley. "Performance changes in champion swimmers aged 30 to 84 years," *Exp. Aging Res.* 10/3 (1984): 141–150.

Johnson, T. "Age-related differences in isometric and dynamic strength and endurance," *Phys. Therapy* 62/7 (1982): 985–989.

Kent, Allegra (with James and Constance Camner). *The dancers' body book.* New York: William Morrow and Company, Inc., 1984.

Kirkland, Gelsey, with Greg Lawrence. *Dancing on my grave.* Garden City, N.Y.: Doubleday & Co., Inc., 1986.

Koegler, Horst. *The concise Oxford dictionary of ballet.* 2nd ed. Oxford: Oxford University Press, 1987.

Kram, M. "Encounter with an athlete," *Sports Illustrated,* September 27, 1971: 93–100.

Lagier, R. "An anatomicopathological approach to the study of articular aging," *Fortschr. Geb. Rontgenstr. Nuklearmed.* 124/6 (1976): 564–570.

Laws, Kenneth. "The physics of dance," *Physics Today* 38/2 (1985): 26.

Lee, Susan A. "Is it the last dance?: Ballet dancers at age 30," *Medical Problems of Performing Artists* March 1988: 27–31.

Lerman, Liz. [Review], *Washington Journal,* March 1988: 1.

Miller, Edward H., Harold J. Schneider, Jeffrey L. Bronson, and David McLain. "A new consideration in athletic injuries," *Clinical Orthopaedica and Related Research* 3 (1975): 181–191.

Myers, Martha. "What dance medicine and science mean to the dancer," in Clarkson, Priscilla M. and Margaret Skrinar, eds. *Science of dance training,* Chapter 1. Champaign, Ill.: Human Kinetics Publishers, Inc., 1988.

Nagrin, Daniel. *How to dance forever: Surviving against the odds.* New York: William Morrow and Co., Inc., 1988.

Novella, Thomas M. "Dancers' shoes and foot care," in Ryan, Allan J. and

Robert E. Stephens, eds. *Dance medicine: A comprehensive guide,* Chapter 10. Chicago: Pluribus Press, Inc./Minneapolis: The Physician and Sports-medicine, 1987.

Orleander, J. and A. Aniansson. "Effect of physical training on skeletal muscle metabolism and ultrastructure in 70- to 75-year-old men," *Acta Physiol. Scand.* 9/2 (1980): 149–154.

Petrofsky, J.S. and A.R. Lind. "Aging, isometric strength and endurance, and cardiovascular responses to static effort," *J. Applied Physiology* 38/1 (1975): 91–95.

Puhl, J., C.H. Brown, and R.O. Voy. *Sports science perspectives for women.* Champaign, Ill.: Human Kinetics Publishers, Inc., 1988.

Rosenberg, Steven L. "Proper footwear for dance for fitness," in Shell, Caroline G., ed. *The dancer as athlete: The 1984 Olympic scientific congress proceedings,* Chapter 14. Champaign, Ill.: Human Kinetics Publishers, Inc., 1986.

Rowe, John W. and Robert L. Kahn. "Human aging: Usual and successful," *Science* 237 (July 10, 1987): 143–149.

Ryan, Allan J. and Robert E. Stephens, eds. *Dance medicine: A comprehensive guide.* Chicago: Pluribus Press, Inc./Minneapolis: The Physician and Sportsmedicine, 1987.

———. *The dancer's complete guide to healthcare and a long career.* Chicago: Bonus Books, 1988.

Schnitt, Jerome M. and Diana Schnitt. "Psychological aspects of dance," in Clarkson, Priscilla M. and Margaret Skrinar, eds. *Science of dance training,* Chapter 13. Champaign, Ill.: Human Kinetics Publishers, Inc., 1988.

———. "Psychological issues in a dancer's career," in Ryan, Allan J. and Robert E. Stephens, eds. *Dance medicine: A comprehensive guide,* Chapter 20. Chicago: Pluribus Press, Inc./Minneapolis: The Physician and Sports-medicine, 1987.

Seals, Jay. "Dance surfaces," in Ryan, Allan J. and Robert E. Stephens, eds. *Dance medicine: A comprehensive guide,* Chapter 19. Chicago: Pluribus Press, Inc./Minneapolis: The Physician and Sportsmedicine, 1987.

Sheehan, George. "Playing the aging game," *The Physician and Sports-medicine* 16/3 (1988): 63.

Shell, Caroline G., ed. *The dancer as athlete: The 1984 Olympic scientific congress proceedings.* Champaign, Ill.: Human Kinetics Publishers, Inc., 1986.

Sommers, Pamela. "Stepping out: Age is a state of mind and body," *The Washington Weekly* (Washington, D.C.), 9 July 1984.

Thomasen, Eivind. *Diseases and injuries of ballet dancers.* Arhus, Denmark: Aarhus Stiftsbogtrykkerie, 1982.

Turner, Jack. "Art and injury: The ABT's Raymond Serrano talks about the agony of ballet," *Massage Therapy Journal* Fall 1988: 20–23.

Vincent, L.M. *Competing with the sylph.* 2nd ed. Princeton, N.J.: Princeton Book Company, Publishers, 1989.

————. *The dancer's book of health.* Princeton, N.J.: Princeton Book Company, Publishers, 1978.

Wallach, Ellen. *Life after performing: Career transitions for dancers* (newsletter and project reports). Lexington, Mass.: Life After Performing, 1988.

Watkins, Andrea and Priscilla M. Clarkson. *Dancing longer, dancing stronger.* Princeton, N.J.: Princeton Book Company, Publishers, 1990.

Wollein, W., N. Bachl, and L. Prokop. "Endurance capacity of trained older aged athletes," *Eur. Heart J.* (5) Suppl. E (November 1984): 21–25.

Wright, Stuart. *Dancer's guide to injuries of the lower extremity.* New York: Cornwall Books, 1985.

Yerg, J.E., D.R. Seals, J.M. Hagberg, and J.O. Holloszy. "Effect of endurance exercise training on ventilatory function in older individuals," *J. Applied Physiology* 58/3 (1985): 791–794.

Zauner, C.W. "Physical fitness in aging men," *Maturitas* 7/3 (1985): 267–271.

Injury and Injury Treatment

Alexander, F.M. *The universal constant in living.* New York: Dutton, 1941.

Arnheim, Daniel D. *Dance injuries: Their prevention and care.* St. Louis: The C.V. Mosby Co., 1980.

Ashley, Merrill. *Dancing for Balanchine.* New York: E.P. Dutton, Inc., 1984.

Bachrach, R.M. "Diagnosis and management of dance injuries to the lower back: An osteopathic approach," Chapter 7 in Shell, Caroline G., ed. *The dancer as athlete: The 1984 Olympic scientific congress proceedings,* Chapter 7. Champaign, Ill.: Human Kinetics Publishers, Inc., 1986.

————. "Injuries to the dancer's spine," in Ryan, Allan J. and Robert E. Stephens, eds. *Dance medicine: A comprehensive guide,* Chapter 13. Chicago: Pluribus Press, Inc./Minneapolis: The Physician and Sportsmedicine, 1987.

Bartenieff, Irmgard, with Dori Lewis. *Body movement: Coping with the environment.* New York: Gordon and Breach, 1980.

Benjamin, Ben. "Creating your own warm-up," *Dance Magazine,* November 1980: 86–88.

Berardi, Gigi. "The agony of dancing," *Los Angeles Times,* May 21, 1989: 61–62.

Cailliet, René. *Understand your backache: A guide to prevention, treatment and relief.* Philadelphia: F.A. Davis Co., 1984.

Clanin, Diana R., Dennis M. Davison, and Janice G. Plastino. "Injury patterns in university dance students," in Shell, Caroline G., ed. *The dancer as athlete: The 1984 Olympic scientific congress proceedings,* Chapter 20. Champaign, Ill.: Human Kinetics Publishers, Inc., 1986.

Clippinger-Robertson, K., Robert S. Hutton, Doris Miller, and T. Richard Nichols. "Mechanical and anatomical factors relating to the incidence and etiology of patellofemoral pain in dancers," in Shell, Caroline G., ed. *The dancer as athlete: The 1984 Olympic scientific congress proceedings,* Chapter 5. Champaign, Ill.: Human Kinetics Publishers, Inc., 1986.

Connolly, Lisa. "Ida Rolf," *Human Behavior* May 1977: 17–23.

Dell, Cecily. *A primer for movement description using Effort-shape and supplementary concepts.* New York: Dance Notation Bureau Press, 1977.

Dolinar, Louis. "Ballet? MD finds it rough as any sport," *The Physician and Sports Medicine* November 1976: 87–92.

Dowd, Irene. "How the dance teacher 'sees,' " *Dance Magazine,* November 1981: 80–81.

Feldenkrais, Moshe. *Awareness through movement.* New York: Harper & Row, Publishers, 1972.

Gantz, Judy. "Evaluation of faulty dance technique patterns: A working model," *Kinesiology and Medicine for Dance* 12/1 (1989): 1–11.

——"Prevention of dance injuries: Evaluation of faulty technique patterns in dance," in *Dance: The study of dance and the place of dance in society,* Proceedings of the VIII Commonwealth and International Conference on Sport, Physical Education, Dance, Recreation and Health, Glasgow, Scotland, July 18–23, 1986.

Glick, F.M. "The female knee in athletics," *The Physician and Sportsmedicine* 2/9 (1973): 35–37.

Gomez, Ninoska. "Moving with somatic awareness: The body-mind centering approach to growth and health," *Journal of Physical Education, Recreation and Dance* September 1988: 90–96.

Gordon, Suzanne. *Off balance: The real world of ballet.* New York: Pantheon Books, 1983.

Hardaker, William T., Lars Erickson, and Martha Myers. "The pathogenesis of dance injury," in Shell, Caroline G., ed. *The dancer as athlete: The 1984 Olympic scientific congress proceedings,* Chapter 2. Champaign, Ill.: Human Kinetics Publishers, Inc., 1986.

Howse, A.J. "Orthopaedists aid ballet," *Clinical Orthopaedics and Related Research* 89 (1972): 52.

Kirkby, Ron. *The probable reality behind structural integration.* La Jolla, Cal.: Rolf Institute of Structural Integration, 1975.

Kirkland, Gelsey, with Greg Lawrence. *Dancing on my Grave.* Garden City, N.Y.: Doubleday & Co., Inc., 1986.

Kleiger, Barnard, "Foot and ankle injuries in dancers," in Ryan, Allan J. and Robert E. Stephens, eds. *Dance medicine: A comprehensive guide,* Chapter 8. Chicago: Pluribus Press, Inc./Minneapolis: The Physician and Sports-medicine, 1987.

Klemp, P., J.E. Stevens, and S. Isaacs. "A hypermobility study in ballet dancers," *J. Rheumatology* 11/5 (1984): 692–696.

Kram, M. "Encounter with an athlete," *Sports Illustrated,* September 27, 1971: 93–100.

Lake, Bernard. "Functional integration—A literal position statement," *Somatics* 4/2 (1983): 12–14.

Lauffenburger, Sandra Kay. "Bartenieff fundamentals: Early detection of potential dance injury," *Journal of Physical Education, Recreation and Dance* May/June 1987: 59–60.

Laws, Kenneth. "Physics and the potential for dance injury," *Medical Problems of Performing Artists* 1/3 (1986): 73–79.

Liemohn, Wendell, Larry B. Snodgrass, and Gina L. Sharpe. "Unresolved controversies in back management—a review," *The Journal of Orthopaedic and Sports Physical Therapy* 9/7 (1988): 239–244.

Micheli, Lyle J. "Back injuries in dancers," *Clinical Journal of Sports Medicine* 2 (1983): 473–484.

———. "Dance injuries: The back, hip and pelvis," in Clarkson, Priscilla M. and Margaret Skrinar, eds. *Science of dance training,* Chapter 10. Champaign, Ill.: Human Kinetics Publishers, Inc., 1988.

Micheli, Lyle J. and Elizabeth R. Micheli. "Back injuries in dancers," in Shell, Caroline G., ed. *The dancer as athlete: The 1984 Olympic scientific congress proceedings,* Chapter 8. Champaign, Ill.: Human Kinetics Publishers, Inc., 1986.

Millar, Anthony P. "Injuries to the neck and upper extremity," in Ryan, Allan J. and Robert E. Stephens, eds. *Dance medicine: A comprehensive guide,* Chapter 14. Chicago: Pluribus Press, Inc./Minneapolis: The Physician and Sportsmedicine, 1987.

Miller, Edward H., Harold J. Schneider, Jeffrey L. Bronson, and David McLain. "A new consideration in athletic injuries," *Clinical Orthopaedica and Related Research* 3 (1975): 181–191.

Minton, Sandra. *Body and self: Partners in movement.* Champaign, Ill.: Human Kinetics Publishers, Inc., 1989.

Molnar, Marika E. "Rehabilitation of the injured dancer," in Ryan, Allan J. and Robert E. Stephens, eds. *Dance medicine: A comprehensive guide,* Chapter 18. Chicago: Pluribus Press, Inc./Minneapolis: The Physician and Sportsmedicine, 1987.

Myers, Martha. "Body therapies and the modern dancer," *Dance Magazine* supplement. New York: Dance Magazine, Inc., 1983.

———. "Perceptual awareness in integrative movement behavior: The role of integrative movement systems (body therapies) in motor performance and expressivity," in Shell, Caroline G., ed. *The dancer as athlete: The 1984 Olympic scientific congress proceedings,* Chapter 17. Champaign, Ill.: Human Kinetics Publishers, Inc., 1986.

———. "What dance medicine and science mean to the dancer," in Clarkson, Priscilla M. and Margaret Skrinar, eds. *Science of dance training,* Chapter 1. Champaign, Ill.: Human Kinetics Publishers, Inc., 1988.

Myers, Martha and Marian Horosko. "When classes are not enough: BODY THERAPIES why, which, and when," *Dance Magazine,* July 1989: 47–51.

Nagrin, Daniel. *How to dance forever: Surviving against the odds.* New York: William Morrow and Co., Inc., 1988.

Nicholas, James A. "Risk factors, sports medicine and the orthopedic system: An overview," *Sports Medicine,* September/October 1975: 243–259.

O'Brien Stillwell, Janet. "The Alexander technique: An innovation for dancers," *Somatics* 4/2 (1983): 15–18.

Powers, J.A. "Characteristic features of injuries of the knees in women," *Clinical Orthopaedic and Related Research* 143 (1979): 120–124.

Puhl, J., C.H. Brown, and R.O. Voy. *Sports science perspectives for women.* Champaign, Ill.: Human Kinetics Publishers, Inc., 1988.

Quirk, R. "Ballet injuries: The Australian experience," *Clinics in Sports Medicine* 2/3 (1983): 507–514.

———. "The dancer's knee," in Ryan, Allan J. and Robert E. Stephens, eds. *Dance medicine: A comprehensive guide,* Chapter 11. Chicago: Pluribus Press, Inc./Minneapolis: The Physician and Sportsmedicine, 1987.

Rosenthal, Eleanor. "Alexander technique: Notes on a teaching method," *Contact Quarterly,* Fall 1981: 14–19.

———. "The Alexander technique—What it is and how it works," *Medical Problems of Performing Artists,* June 1987: 53–57.

Rovere, G.D., L.X. Webb, A.G. Gristina, and J.M. Vogel. "Musculoskeletal injuries in threatrical dance students," *American Journal of Sports Medicine* 11 (1983): 195–198.

Ryan, Allan J. and Robert E. Stephens. *The dancer's complete guide to healthcare and a long career.* Chicago: Bonus Books, 1988.

————. "The epidemiology of dance injuries," in Ryan, Allan J. and Robert E. Stephens, eds. *Dance medicine: A comprehensive guide,* Chapter 1. Chicago: Pluribus Press, Inc./Minneapolis: The Physician and Sportsmedicine, 1987.

Safran, M.R., W.E. Garrett, and A.V. Seaber. "The role of warmup in muscular injury prevention," *American Journal of Sports Medicine* 16 (1988): 123–129.

Sammarco, G.J. "The dancer's hip," in Ryan, Allan J. and Robert E. Stephens, eds. *Dance medicine: A comprehensive guide,* Chapter 12. Chicago: Pluribus Press, Inc./Minneapolis: The Physician and Sportsmedicine, 1987.

Sammarco, G.J. and E.H. Miller. "Forefoot conditions in dancers: Part I," *Foot and Ankle* 3/2 (1982): 85–92.

Seals, J. "Dance surfaces," in Ryan, Allan J. and Robert E. Stephens, eds. *Dance medicine: A comprehensive guide,* Chapter 19. Chicago: Pluribus Press, Inc./Minneapolis: The Physician and Sportsmedicine, 1987.

Shaw, J. "The nature, frequency and patterns of dance injuries: A survey of college dance students," unpublished M.A. thesis, University of Utah, 1977.

Shell, Caroline G., ed. *The dancer as athlete: The 1984 Olympic scientific congress proceedings.* Champaign, Ill.: Human Kinetics Publishers, Inc., 1986.

Skinner, Joan, Bridget Davis, Sally Metcalf, and Kris Wheeler. "Notes on the Skinner releasing technique," *Contact Quarterly,* Fall 1979: 8–13.

Solomon, Ruth and Lyle Micheli. "Concepts in the prevention of dance injuries: A survey and analysis," in Shell, Caroline G., ed. *The dancer as athlete: The 1984 Olympic scientific congress proceedings,* Chapter 21. Champaign, Ill.: Human Kinetics Publishers, Inc., 1986.

Solomon, Ruth, Sandra C. Minton, and John Solomon, eds. *Preventing dance injuries: An interdisciplinary perspective.* Reston, Va.: AAHPERD, 1990.

Stephens, Robert E. "The etiology of injuries in ballet," in Ryan, Allan J. and Robert E. Stephens, eds. *Dance medicine: A comprehensive guide,* Chapter 2. Chicago: Pluribus Press, Inc./Minneapolis: The Physician and Sportsmedicine, 1987.

Sweigard, Lulu E. *Human movement potential: Its ideokinetic facilitation.* New York: Harper & Row, Publishers, 1974.

Teitz, Carol C. "First aid, immediate care, and rehabilitation of knee and ankle injuries in dancers and **athletes**," in Shell, Caroline G., ed. *The dancer as athlete: The 1984 Olympic scientific congress proceedings*, Chapter 6. Champaign, Ill.: Human Kinetics Publishers, Inc., 1986.

Thomasen, Eivind. *Diseases and injuries of ballet dancers.* Arhus, Denmark: Aarhus Stiftsbogtrykkerie, 1982.

———— "The loose metatarsophalangeal joint in dancers," in Ryan, Allan J. and Robert E. Stephens, eds. *Dance medicine: A comprehensive guide*, Chapter 8. Chicago: Pluribus Press, Inc./Minneapolis: The Physician and Sportsmedicine, 1987.

Tinbergen, Nikolaas. "Ethology and stress diseases," *Science* 185 (5 July 1974): 20–27.

Vincent, L.M. *Competing with the sylph.* 2nd ed. Princeton: Princeton Book Company, Publishers, 1989.

————. *The dancer's book of health.* Princeton: Princeton Book Company, Publishers, 1978.

Washington, E.L. "The emergence of sports medicine and dance medicine as an important field of study," in Shell, Caroline G., ed. *The dancer as athlete: The 1984 Olympic scientific congress proceedings*, Chapter 1. Champaign, Ill.: Human Kinetics Publishers, Inc., 1986.

————. "Musculoskeletal injuries in theatrical dancers: Site, frequency and severity," *American Journal of Sports Medicine* 6/2 (1978): 75–98.

————. "Musculoskeletal problems in modern, jazz and 'show biz' dancers," in Ryan, Allan J. and Robert E. Stephens, eds. *Dance medicine: A comprehensive guide*, Chapter 15. Chicago: Pluribus Press, Inc./Minneapolis: The Physician and Sportsmedicine, 1987.

Weiker, Gordon G. "Dance injuries: The knee, ankle and foot," in Clarkson, Priscilla M. and Margaret Skrinar, eds. *Science of dance training*, Chapter 9. Champaign, Ill.: Human Kinetics Publishers, Inc., 1988.

Wing, Heather. "Rolfing movement integration: Movement education for everyday life," *Somatics* 4/2 (1983): 19–24.

Wright, Stuart. *Dancer's guide to injuries of the lower extremity.* New York: Cornwall Books, 1985.

Technique and Training

Bachrach, R.M. "Diagnosis and management of dance injuries to the lower back: An osteopathic approach," in Shell, Caroline G., ed. *The dancer as athlete: The 1984 Olympic scientific congress proceedings*, Chapter 7. Champaign, Ill.: Human Kinetics Publishers, Inc., 1986.

Blasis, Carlo. *An elementary treatise upon the theory and practice of the art of dancing*. Reprint. New York: Dover, 1968.

Cailliet, Rene. *Understand your backache: A guide to prevention, treatment and relief*. Philadelphia: F.A. Davis Co., 1984.

Chmelar, Robin D., Barry Shultz, Robert Ruhling, Sally Fitt, and Mary Johnson. "Isokinetic characteristics of the knee in female, professional and university, ballet and modern dancers," *The Journal of Orthopaedic and Sports Physical Therapy* 9/12 (1988): 410–418.

Clanin, Diana R., Dennis M. Davison, and Janice G. Plastino. "Injury patterns in university dance students," in Shell, Caroline G., ed. *The dancer as athlete: The 1984 Olympic scientific congress proceedings*, Chapter 20. Champaign, Ill.: Human Kinetics Publishers, Inc., 1986.

Clippinger-Robertson, Karen. "Flexibility in dance," *Kinesiology and Medicine for Dance* 12/2 (1990): 1–16.

———. "Principles of dance training," in Clarkson, Priscilla M. and Margaret Skrinar, eds. *Science of dance training*, Chapter 5. Champaign, Ill.: Human Kinetics Publishers, Inc., 1988.

Clippinger-Robertson, Karen, Robert S. Hutton, Doris Miller, and T. Richard Nichols. "Mechanical and anatomical factors relating to the incidence and etiology of patellofemoral pain in dancers," in Shell, Caroline G., ed. *The dancer as athlete: The 1984 Olympic scientific congress proceedings*, Chapter 5. Champaign, Ill.: Human Kinetics Publishers, Inc., 1986.

Fitt, Sally Sevey. *Dance kinesiology*. New York: Schirmer Books, 1988.

Galea, V. and R.W. Norman. "Bone-on-bone forces at the ankle joint during a rapid dynamic movement," in Winter, D., ed. *Biomechanics IX A*, pp. 71–76. Champaign, Ill.: Human Kinetics Publishers, Inc., 1985.

Gantz, Judy. "Evaluation of faulty dance technique patterns: A working model," *Kinesiology and Medicine for Dance* 12/1 (1989): 1–11.

———"Prevention of dance injuries: Evaluation of faulty technique patterns in dance," *Dance: The study of dance and the place of dance in society*. Proceedings of the VIII Commonwealth and International Conference on Sport, Physical Education, Dance, Recreation and Health, Glasgow, Scotland, July 18–23, 1986.

Hardaker, William T., Lars Erickson, and Martha Myers. "The pathogenesis of dance injury," in Shell, Caroline G., ed. *The dancer as athlete: The 1984 Olympic scientific congress proceedings*, Chapter 2. Champaign, Ill.: Human Kinetics Publishers, Inc., 1986.

Hays, J.P. *Modern dance: A biomechanical approach to teaching*. St. Louis: C.V. Mosby, 1981.

Hinson, M.M. *Kinesiology*. Dubuque, Iowa: Wm. C. Brown, 1977.

Hinson, M., S. Buckman, J. Tate, and C. Sherrill. "The grand jeté en tournant entrelacé (tour jeté): An analysis through motion photography," *Dance Research Journal* 10 (1978): 9–13.

Howse, A.J. "The young ballet dancer," in Ryan, Allan J. and Robert E. Stephens, eds. *Dance medicine: A comprehensive guide*, Chapter 7. Chicago: Pluribus Press, Inc./Minneapolis: The Physician and Sportsmedicine, 1987.

Kleiger, Barnard. "Foot and ankle injuries in dancers," in Ryan, Allan J. and Robert E. Stephens, eds. *Dance medicine: A comprehensive guide*, Chapter 8. Chicago: Pluribus Press, Inc./Minneapolis: The Physician and Sportsmedicine, 1987.

Klemp, P., J.E. Stevens, and S. Isaacs. "A hypermobility study in ballet dancers," *J. Rheumatology* 11/5 (1984): 692–696.

Kneeland, A. "The dancer prepares," *Dance Magazine*, March–June 1966: 49–53; 57–59; 65–66; 67–69.

Kravitz, S.R., C.J. Murgia, S. Huber, K. Fink, M. Shaffer, and L. Varela. "Bunion deformity and the forces generated around the great toe: A biomechanical approach to analysis of pointe dance, classical ballet," in Shell, Caroline G., ed. *The dancer as athlete: The 1984 Olympic scientific congress proceedings*, Chapter 22. Champaign, Ill.: Human Kinetics Publishers, Inc., 1986.

Laws, Kenneth. "Physics and ballet: A new *pas de deux*," in D.T. Taplin, ed. *New directions in dance*, pp. 137–146. New York: Pergamon, 1979.

———. "Physics and the potential for dance injury," *Medical Problems of Performing Artists* 1/3 (1986): 73–79.

———. "The physics of dance," *Physics Today* 38/2 (1985): 26.

Lei, Li with Kenneth Laws. "The physical analysis of *Da She Yan Tiao*," *Kinesiology for Dance* 11/4 (1989): 9–11.

Lycholat, T. "Lifting techniques in dance: A scientific investigation," *Dancing Times* 73 (1982): 123 ff.

Micheli, L. J. "Back injuries in dancers," *Clinical Journal of Sports Medicine* 2 (1983): 473–484.

———. "Dance injuries: The back, hip and pelvis," in Clarkson, Priscilla M. and Margaret Skrinar, eds. *Science of dance training*, Chapter 10. Champaign, Ill.: Human Kinetics Publishers, Inc., 1988.

Micheli, Lyle J. and Elizabeth R. Micheli. "Back injuries in dancers," in Shell, Caroline G., ed. *The dancer as athlete: The 1984 Olympic scientific congress proceedings*, Chapter 8. Champaign, Ill.: Human Kinetics Publishers, Inc., 1986.

Micheli, Lyle J. and Ruth Solomon. "Training the young dancer," in Ryan, Allan J. and Robert E. Stephens, eds. *Dance medicine: A comprehensive guide*, Chapter 3. Chicago: Pluribus Press, Inc./Minneapolis: The Physician and Sportsmedicine, 1987.

Millar, Anthony P. "Injuries to the neck and upper extremity," in Ryan, Allan J. and Robert E. Stephens, eds. *Dance medicine: A comprehensive guide*, Chapter 14. Chicago: Pluribus Press, Inc./Minneapolis: The Physician and Sportsmedicine, 1987.

Molnar, Marika E. "Rehabilitation of the injured dancer," in Ryan, Allan J. and Robert E. Stephens, eds. *Dance medicine: A comprehensive guide*, Chapter 18. Chicago: Pluribus Press, Inc./Minneapolis: The Physician and Sportsmedicine, 1987.

Myers, Martha. "What dance medicine and science mean to the dancer," in Clarkson, Priscilla M. and Margaret Skrinar, eds. *Science of dance training*, Chapter 1. Champaign, Ill.: Human Kinetics Publishers, Inc., 1988.

Powers, J.A. "Characteristic features of injuries of the knees in women," *Clinical Orthopaedic and Related Research* 143 (1979): 120–124.

Puhl, J., C.H. Brown, and R.O. Voy. *Sports science perspectives for women*. Champaign, Ill.: Human Kinetics Publishers, Inc., 1988.

Quirk, R. "Ballet injuries: The Australian experience," *Clinics in Sports Medicine* 2/3 (1983): 507–514.

————. "The dancer's knee," in Ryan, Allan J. and Robert E. Stephens, eds. *Dance medicine: A comprehensive guide*, Chapter 11. Chicago: Pluribus Press, Inc./Minneapolis: The Physician and Sportsmedicine, 1987.

Ranney, Donald. "Biomechanics of dance," in Clarkson, Priscilla M. and Margaret Skrinar, eds. *Science of dance training*, Chapter 8. Champaign, Ill.: Human Kinetics Publishers, Inc., 1988.

Ryan, Allan J. and Robert E. Stephens. *The dancer's complete guide to healthcare and a long career*. Chicago: Bonus Books, 1988.

————. "The epidemiology of dance injuries," in Ryan, Allan J. and Robert E. Stephens, eds. *Dance medicine: A comprehensive guide*, Chapter 1. Chicago: Pluribus Press, Inc./Minneapolis: The Physician and Sportsmedicine, 1987.

Ryman, R.S. "A kinematic analysis of selected *grand allegro* jumps," *Dance Research Annual* 9 (1978): 231–242.

Ryman, R.S. and D.A. Ranney. "A preliminary investigation of skeletal and muscular action in the *grand battement devant*," *Dance Research Journal* 11/1–2 (1978–79): 2–11.

Sammarco, G.J. "The dancer's hip," in Ryan, Allan J. and Robert E. Stephens, eds. *Dance medicine: A comprehensive guide*, Chapter 12.

Chicago: Pluribus Press, Inc./Minneapolis: The Physician and Sports-medicine, 1987.

Sammarco, G.J. and E.H. Miller. "Forefoot conditions in dancers: Part I," *Foot and Ankle* 3/2 (1982): 85–92.

Skrinar, Margaret. "Selected motor learning applications to the technique class," in Clarkson, Priscilla M. and Margaret Skrinar, eds. *Science of dance training*, Chapter 14. Champaign, Ill.: Human Kinetics Publishers, Inc., 1988.

Solomon, Ruth and Lyle Micheli. "Concepts in the prevention of dance injuries: A survey and analysis," in Shell, Caroline G., ed. *The dancer as athlete: The 1984 Olympic scientific congress proceedings*, Chapter 21. Champaign, Ill.: Human Kinetics Publishers, Inc., 1986.

Stephens, Robert E. "The etiology of injuries in ballet," in Ryan, Allan J. and Robert E. Stephens, eds. *Dance medicine: A comprehensive guide*, Chapter 2. Chicago: Pluribus Press, Inc./Minneapolis: The Physician and Sports-medicine, 1987.

Watkins, Andrea and Priscilla Clarkson. *Dancing longer, dancing stronger.* Princeton: Princeton Book Company, Publishers, 1990.

Weiker, Gordon G. "Dance injuries: The knee, ankle and foot," in Clarkson, Priscilla M. and Margaret Skrinar, eds. *Science of dance training*, Chapter 9. Champaign, Ill.: Human Kinetics Publishers, Inc., 1988.

Wright, Stuart. *Dancer's guide to injuries of the lower extremity.* New York: Cornwall Books, 1985.

The Fit Dancer: Conditioning for Strength, Endurance, and Flexibility

Alter, Judy. *Stretch and strengthen.* Boston: Houghton Mifflin Co., 1986.

————. *Surviving exercise.* Boston: Houghton Mifflin Co., 1983.

Alter, Michael J. *Science of stretching.* Champaign, Ill.: Human Kinetics Publishers, Inc., 1988.

Chatfield, Steven and William C. Byrnes. "Cardiovascular aspects of dance," in Clarkson, Priscilla M. and Margaret Skrinar, eds. *Science of dance training*, Chapter 6. Champaign, Ill.: Human Kinetics Publishers, Inc., 1988.

Chmelar, Robin D., Barry Shultz, Robert Ruhling, Sally Fitt, and Mary Johnson. "Isokinetic characteristics of the knee in female, professional and university, ballet and modern dancers," *The Journal of Orthopaedic and Sports Physical Therapy* 9/12 (1988): 410–418.

Clarkson, Priscilla M. "Energy production in dance," in Clarkson, Priscilla

M. and Margaret Skrinar, eds. *Science of dance training*, Chapter 4. Champaign, Ill.: Human Kinetics Publishers, Inc., 1988.

Clarkson, P.M., P.S. Freedson, B. Keller, D. Carney, and M. Skrinar. "Maximal oxygen uptake, nutritional patterns and body composition of adolescent female ballet dancers," *Research Quarterly for Exercise and Sport* 56 (1985): 180–184.

Clippinger-Robertson, Karen. "Components of an aerobic dance-exercise class," in *Aerobic dance-exercise instructor manual*, Chapter 5. San Diego: IDEA Foundation, 1987.

──────. "Flexibility in dance," *Kinesiology and Medicine for Dance* 12/2 (1990): 1–16.

──────. "Principles of dance training," in Clarkson, Priscilla M. and Margaret Skrinar, eds. *Science of dance training*, Chapter 5. Champaign, Ill.: Human Kinetics Publishers, Inc., 1988.

Cohen, Jerald L. "The cardiovascular and metabolic demands of classical dance," in Ryan, Allan J. and Robert E. Stephens, eds. *Dance medicine: A comprehensive guide*, Chapter 4. Chicago: Pluribus Press, Inc./Minneapolis: The Physician and Sportsmedicine, 1987.

Cohen, J.L., P.K. Gupta, E. Lichistein, and K.D. Chadda. "The heart of a dancer: Noninvasive cardiac evaluation of professional ballet dancers," *American Journal of Cardiology* 45 (1980): 959–965.

Cohen, J.L., K.R. Segal, I. Witriol, and W.D. McArdle. "Cardiorespiratory responses to ballet exercise and the VO_2max of elite ballet dancers," *Medicine and Science in Sports and Exercise* 14 (1982): 212–217.

Davidson, Dennis M. "Dance and cardiorespiratory fitness," in Shell, Caroline G., ed. *The dancer as athlete: The 1984 Olympic scientific congress proceedings*, Chapter 13. Champaign, Ill.: Human Kinetics Publishers, Inc., 1986.

DeGuzman, J.A. "Dance as a contributor to cardiovascular fitness and alteration of body composition," *Journal of Physical Education and Recreation* 50 (1979): 88–91.

De Vries, Herbert A. "Evaluation of static stretching procedures for improvement of flexibility," *Research Quarterly for Exercise and Sport* 33 (1962): 222–229.

Garhammer, John. *Sports Illustrated strength training*. New York: Harper & Row, 1986.

Holt, L.E., T.M. Travis, and T. Okita. "Comparative study of three stretching techniques," *Perceptual and Motor Skills* 31 (1970): 611–616.

Hortobagyi, T., J. Faludi, J. Tihanyi, and B. Merkeley. "Effects of intense 'stretching'-flexibility training on the mechanical profile of the knee extensors and on the range of motion of the hip joint," *Int. Journal Sport Med.* 6 (1985): 317–321.

Kabat, H. "Proprioceptive facilitation in therapeutic exercise," in S. Licht, ed. *Therapeutic exercise.* New Haven, Conn.: Williams and Wilkins, 1965.

Kasch, F.W. and J.P. Wallace. "Physiological variables during 10 years of endurance exercise," *Med. Sci. Sports* 8/1 (1976): 5–8.

Katch, Frank I. and William D. McArdle. *Nutrition, weight control, and exercise.* 2nd ed. Philadelphia: Lea & Febiger, 1983; 3rd ed., 1988.

Kent, Allegra, with James and Constance Camner. *The dancers' body book.* New York: William Morrow and Company, Inc., 1984.

Kirkendall, D.T. and L.H. Calabrese. "Physiological aspects of dance," *Clin. Sports Med.* 2/3 (1983): 525–537.

Liemohn, W. "Flexibility and muscular strength," *Journal of Physical Education, Recreation and Dance,* September 1988: 37–40.

Lubell, Adele. "Potentially dangerous exercises: Are they harmful to all?" *Phys. Sportsmed.* 17/1 (1989): 187–192.

Puhl, J., C.H. Brown, and R.O. Voy. *Sports science perspectives for women.* Champaign, Ill.: Human Kinetics Publishers, Inc., 1988.

Ryan, Allan J. and Robert E. Stephens. *The dancer's complete guide to healthcare & a long career.* Chicago: Bonus Books, 1988.

Selye, H. *Stress without distress.* New York: J.P. Lippincott, 1974.

Sharkey, Brian J. *Physiology of Fitness.* 2nd ed. Champaign, Ill.: Human Kinetics Publishers, Inc., 1984.

Watkins, Andrea and Priscilla Clarkson. *Dancing longer, dancing stronger.* Princeton, N.J.: Princeton Book Company, Publishers, 1990.

Wolkodoff, Neil E. "Physiology and application of flexibility programs," paper presented at the IDEA One-to-One Fitness Conference, Los Angeles, California, April 14–16, 1989.

Nutrition and Diet

AHA (American Heart Association). *Heart cuisine.* Los Angeles, Cal.: AHA, undated.

Bell, Douglas G. and Ira Jacobs. "Muscle fiber-specific glycogen utilization in strength-trained males and females," *Medicine and Science in Sports and Exercise* 21/6 (1989): 649–654.

Benson, Joan E., Donna M. Gillien, Kathy Bourdet, and Alvin R. Loosli. "Inadequate nutrition and chronic calorie restriction in adolescent ballerinas," *The Physician and Sportsmedicine* 13/10 (1985): 79–90.

————. "Nutritional considerations for ballet dancers," in Clarkson, Priscilla M. and Margaret Skrinar, eds. *Science of dance training,* Chapter 12. Champaign, Ill.: Human Kinetics Publishers, Inc., 1988.

Bonbright, Jane M. "The nutritional status of female ballet dancers 15–18 years of age," *Dance Research Journal* 21/2 (1989): 9–14.

Bright-See, E., J. Croy, J. Bradshaw, D.A. Pearce, D.J. Secker, and L. Yoneyama. "Nutrition beliefs and practices of ballet students," *Journal of the Canadian Dietetic Association* 39/4 (1978): 324–331.

Brody, Jane E. "Jane Brody's *The New York Times* guide to personal health" (1982), in Berardi, Gigi M., ed. *World Food, Population and Development,* Chapter 32. Totowa, N.J.: Rowman and Allanheld, 1985.

Brotherhood, J.R. "Nutrition and sports performance," *Sports Med.,* Sept.–Oct. 1984: 350–389.

Burckes-Miller, Mardie and David R. Black. "Eating disorders: A problem in athletics?" *Health Education,* February/March 1988: 22–25.

Calabrese, L.H., D.T. Kirkendall, M. Floyd, S. Rapoport, G.W. Williams, G.G. Weiker, and J.A. Bergfield. "Menstrual abnormalities, nutritional patterns, and body composition in female classical dancers," *The Physician and Sportsmedicine* 11/2 (1983): 86–98.

Chmelar, Robin D. and Sally Fitt. *Dancing at your peak: Diet.* Princeton, N.J.: Princeton Book Company, Publishers, 1990.

Clark, Nancy. "How to increase calorie intake," *The Physician and Sportsmedicine* 16/6 (1988): 140.

Clarkson, Priscilla M. "Energy production in dance," in Clarkson, Priscilla M. and Margaret Skrinar, eds. *Science of dance training,* Chapter 4. Champaign, Ill.: Human Kinetics Publishers, Inc., 1988.

Clarkson, P.M., P.S. Freedson, B. Keller, D. Carney, and M. Skrinar. "Maximal oxygen uptake, nutritional patterns and body composition of adolescent female ballet dancers," *Research Quarterly for Exercise and Sport* 56 (1985): 180–184.

Cohen, J.L., L. Potosnak, O. Frank, and H. Baker. "A nutritional and hematologic assessment of elite ballet dancers," *The Physician and Sportsmedicine* 13/5 (1985): 43–54.

Coleman, Ellen. "Nutrition and weight control," in *Aerobic dance-exercise instructor manual,* Chapter 3. San Diego: IDEA Foundation, 1987.

Hamilton, E.M., E.N. Whitney, and F.S. Sizer. *Nutrition: Concepts and controversies.* 3rd ed. St. Paul, Minn.: West Publishing Co., 1985.

Hamilton, L.H., J. Brooks-Gunn, and M.P. Warren. "Nutritional intake of female dancers: A reflection of eating problems," *International Journal of Eating Disorders* 5 (1986): 925–934.

Heaney, R.P., J.C. Gallagher, C.C. Johnston, R. Neer, A.M. Parfitt, and G.D. Whedon. "Calcium nutrition and bone health in the elderly," *Am. J. Clin. Nut.*, November 1982 (3615 Suppl.): 986–1013.

Jacobson, P.C., W. Beaver, S.A. Grubb, T.N. Taft, and R.V. Talmadge. "Bone density in women: College athletes and older athletic women," *J. Orthop. Res.* 2/4 (1984): 328–332.

Johnston, C.C. and C. Slemenda. "Osteoporosis—an overview," *The Physician and Sportsmedicine* 15/11 (1987): 64–68.

Kanders, B., D.W. Dempster, and R. Lindsay. "Interaction of calcium nutrition and physical activity on bone mass in young women," *J. Bone Mineral Research* 3/2 (1988): 145–149.

Katch, Frank I. and William D. McArdle. *Nutrition, weight control, and exercise*, 2nd ed. Philadelphia: Lea & Febiger, 1983; 3rd ed., 1988.

Kent, Allegra, with James and Constance Camner. *The dancers' body book.* New York: William Morrow and Company, Inc., 1984.

Kvasova, A.P. "Evaluation of a balanced diet for students at a ballet school," *Higiena Sanitariya* 8 (1974): 27–29.

Lane, N., W. Bevier, M. Bouxsein, R. Wiswell, D. Carter, and R. Marcus. "Effect of exercise intensity on bone mineral," paper presented at the American College of Sports Medicine Annual Meeting, Dallas, Texas, May 1988.

Lappé, Frances Moore. *Diet for a small planet.* New York: Ballantine Books, 1971.

Latham, Michael. "Nutrition and infection in national development" (1975), in Berardi, Gigi M., ed. *World food, population and development,* Chapter 34. Totowa, N.J.: Rowman and Allanheld, 1985.

Lindquist, O., C. Bengtsson, T. Hansson, and B. Rovs. "Bone mineral content in relation to age and menopause in middle-aged women," *Scand. J. Clin. Lab. Invest.* 41/3 (1981): 215–223.

Lindsay, Robert. "Estrogens and osteoporosis," *The Physician and Sportsmedicine* 15/11 (1988): 105–108.

Loosli, Alvin R., Joan Benson, and Donna M. Gillien. "Nutrition and the dancer," in Ryan, Allan J. and Robert E. Stephens, eds. *Dance medicine: A comprehensive guide,* Chapter 6. Chicago: Pluribus Press, Inc./Minneapolis: The Physician and Sportsmedicine, 1987.

Mazes, R.B. "On aging bone loss," *Clin. Orthop.* 165 (1982): 239–252.

McCarthy, Paul. "How much protein do athletes really need?" *The Physician and Sportsmedicine* 17/5 (1989): 170–175.

Mole, Paul A., Judith S. Stern, Cynthia L. Schultz, Edmund M. Bernauer, and Bryan J. Holcomb. "Exercise reverses depressed metabolic rate produced by severe caloric restriction," *Medicine and Science in Sports and Exercise* 2/1 (1989): 29–33.

Munnings, Frances. "Exercise and estrogen in women's health: getting a clearer picture," *The Physician and Sportsmedicine* 16/5 (1988): 152–161.

National Research Council. *Recommended dietary allowances.* 9th ed. Washington, D.C.: National Academy Press, 1980; 10th ed., 1989.

"Overcoming the ten-pound obsession," *Tufts University Diet and Nutrition Letter* 6/11 (1988): 3–6.

Poehlman, Eric T. "A review: Exercise and its influence on resting energy metabolism in man," *Medicine and Science in Sports and Exercise* 21/5 (1989): 515–525.

Rosen, Lionel W. and David O. Hough. "Pathogenic weight-control behaviors of female college gymnasts," *The Physician and Sportsmedicine* 16/9 (1988): 141–146.

Rutherford, O.M., A.M. Mayer, D.A. Jones, and M. Nelson. "Physical activity and bone mass in women aged 35–40," paper presented at the American College of Sports Medicine Annual Meeting, Dallas, Texas, May 1988.

Sedlock, Darlene A., Jean A. Fissinger, and Christopher L. Melby. "Effect of exercise intensity and duration on postexercise energy expenditure," *Medicine and Science in Sports and Exercise* 21/6 (1989): 662–668.

Slavin, Joanne L., Greg Lanners, and Mark A. Engstrom. "Amino acid supplements: Beneficial or risky?" *The Physician and Sportsmedicine* 16/3 (1988): 221–224.

Smith, D.M., M.R. Khairi, J. Norton, and C.C. Johnston, Jr. "Age and activity effects on rate of bone mineral loss," *J. Clin. Invest.* 58/3 (1976): 716–721.

Smith, Everett L. and Catherine Gilligan. "Effects of inactivity and exercise on bone," *The Physician and Sportsmedicine* 15/11 (1987): 91–100.

Smith, E.L and D.M. Raab. "Osteoporosis and physical activity," *Acta Med. Scand.* 711 (1986): 149–156.

Stamford, Bryant. "Meals and the timing of exercise," *The Physician and Sportsmedicine* 17/11 (1989): 151.

Stillman, R.J., B.H. Massey, R.A. Boileau, and M.H. Slaughter. "Physical activity and bone mineral in women," paper presented at the American College of Sports Medicine Annual Meeting, Dallas, Texas, May 1988.

Van Itallie, T.B. and M. Yang. "Current concepts in nutrition: Diet and weight loss," *New England Journal of Medicine* 297 (1977): 1158–1161.

Vincent, Larry, M. *Competing with the sylph.* 2nd ed. Princeton, N.J.: Princeton Book Company, Publishers, 1989.

Wallberg-Henriksson, Harriet. "Acute exercise: Fuel homeostasis and glucose transport in insulin-dependent diabetes mellitus," *Medicine and Science in Sports and Exercise* 21/4 (1989): 356–361.

White, L.A. "Nutritional intake, percent body fat, and physical fitness among professional ballerinas," unpublished master's thesis, University of Utah, 1982.

Wurts, M.K. and D.A. Lally. "Exercise and bone mineral content in pre- and postmenopausal women," paper presented at the American College of Sports Medicine Annual Meeting, Dallas, Texas, May 1988.

Index

Italicized numbers indicate illustrations.

265

Center of gravity, weight shifts from, 105
Central nervous system, energy source, 160, 174, 175
Central Pennsylvania Youth Ballet (CPYB), 95
Certified Movement Analysts (C.M.A.s), 38
Chair stepping, 141
Chatfield, Steven, 137
Childs, Lucinda, 135
Chiropractors, 38
Chloride, 174
Chmelar, Robin, 141; exercise program, 120–30
Cholesterol, 161
Choreography: aerobic, 135; dangerous, 193–94, 241n54; Grossman and, 28–29; and overuse injuries, 9; for self, 194–98, 202–3
Chromium, 174
Chronic tendinitis, 51
Clippinger-Robertson, Karen, 84, 86, 97, 150; and training programs, 109–10
Combinations, movement, 134
Competing with the Sylph, Vincent, 17–19
Complete proteins, 163
Complex carbohydrates, 160, 172, 174, 177
Compression fractures, 34–35
Compressive strain syndrome, 56
Conditioning, 97–151, 237n18; Caras and, 186
Conscious control, Alexander technique, 46–47
Conservative treatment of injury, 50
Constructive rest position, 45
Contraction, Graham technique, 69
Contracts. *See* Union contracts
Control, dancers and, 188–201
Coordination, 97; flexibility and, 142
Copper, 174; adult RDA, 170
Coracobrachialis exercises, *127,* 128
Corbin, Patrick, 228n8
Corps dancers, 188; and injuries, 6
Correct movement, 69–70; anatomical variations and, 80–86; vertical lift, *77, 79*
Corrective devices, 51, *52*
Cortisone injections, 53

Cotillon, Balanchine, 6
CPYB. *See* Central Pennsylvania Youth Ballet
Cross-country skiing, 141
Cruz, Mirabel, *100*
Cryotherapy, 35–36
Cunningham, Merce, *21, 58,* 92
Cybex machines, 237n18; training program, 120–28, *121, 123–27*
Cycling, 140

D, vitamin, adult RDA, 167
Daily body work, Karipides program, 101–8, *102–4*
Daily caloric intake of dancers, 159
Dance companies, performance schedules, 5
Dance medicine, 4
Dance movements. *See* Movement
Dancer's heel, 33
Dancers of the Third Age, 190, *191*
Dancers' union, 199–201
Dancing for Balanchine, Ashley, 61
Dean, Laura, 135
Deficiencies, dietary, 171–72, 174
Dehydration, 164–65
de Lavallade, Carmen, 20, 196, *197*
Demands, professional, 3–4
Demi-plié, *71, 83,* 84; second position, rolling in of feet, *82*
de Ribère, Lisa, 95
De Vries, Herbert A., 144
Diet, 174–82. *See also* Nutrition
Dietary fiber, 160, 173
Dietary-induced thermogenesis, 165
Dieting: Caras and, 186–87; obsessive, 179–80, 182
Disaccharides, 160
Diuretics, 17
Dowd, Irene, 45
Duell, Daniel, 100, *153,* 153–54
Duncan, Jeff, *205,* 205–6
Duration: for aerobic training, 139; of dance movements, 134; of stretching exercises, 147
Dynamic alignment, Myers and, 43

E, vitamin, adult RDA, 167
EAAs. *See* Essential Amino Acids
Eagle machines, 120
Eating disorders, 17, 158, 184
Edgerton, Glenn, 6, 98, *99,* 228n8

Profile Credits

Murray Louis
Photo by Tom Caravaglia

Patricia McBride and Adam Lüders
Photo courtesy © Steven Caras, 1990

Danny Grossman
Photo by Cylla von Tiedemann
Courtesy of the Danny Grossman Dance Company

Daniel Nagrin
Photo by Phyllis Steele

Merrill Ashley
Photo courtesy © Steven Caras, 1990

Patricia McBride and Adam Lüders
Photo courtesy © Steven Caras, 1990

Risa Steinberg
Photo © Johan Elbers, 1990

Erick Hawkins
Photo by Daniel Kramer
Courtesy of the Erick Hawkins Dance Company

June Finch
Photo by Jed Downhill

Jan Hyatt and Kelly Holt
Photo by Bill Owen

Kenneth Laws
Photo by Tom Wilson
Courtesy of *The Dickinsonian*, Dickinson College

Kathryn Karipides with Kelly Holt in *Reflections*
Photo © 1976 by James Fry

Daniel Duell with Heather Watts
Photo courtesy © Steven Caras, 1990

Jan Hyatt and Kelly Holt
Photo by Bill Owen

Keith Sabado
Photo courtesy of Monnaie Dance Group/Mark Morris

Judith Fugate
Photo courtesy © Steven Caras, 1990

Steven Caras rehearsing Maribel Modrono and Fabrizio Betti of
the Miami City Ballet
Photo courtesy © Leslie Sternlieb, 1990

Wendy Perron
Photo © Johan Elbers, 1990

Christine Spizzo
Photo by Gilles Larrain

Jeff Duncan
Photo courtesy of Dance Theatre Workshop